HEALTH AND RISK COMMUNICATION

Health and Risk Communication provides a critical and comprehensive overview of the core issues surrounding health and risk communication from the perspective of applied linguistics. It outlines the ways applied linguistics differs from other methods of understanding health and risk communication, assesses the benefits and limitations of the approaches used by different scholars in the field, and offers an innovative framework for consolidating past research and charting new directions.

Utilizing data from clinical interactions and everyday life, this book addresses a number of crucial questions including:

- How are the everyday actions we take around health constructed and constrained through discourse?
- What is the role of texts in influencing health behaviour, and how are these texts put together and interpreted by readers?
- How are actions and identities around health and risk negotiated in situated social interactions, and what are the factors that influence these negotiations?
- How will new technologies like genetic screening influence the way we communicate about health?
- How does communication about health and risk help create communities and institutions and reflect and reproduce broader ideologies and patterns of power and inequality within societies?

Health and Risk Communication: An Applied Linguistic Perspective is essential reading for advanced students and researchers studying and working in this area.

Rodney H. Jones is Associate Professor of English at City University of Hong Kong.

HEALTH AND RISK COMMUNICATION

An Applied Linguistic Perspective

Rodney H. Jones

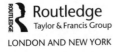

Routledge
Taylor & Francis Group

LONDON AND NEW YORK

First published 2013
by Routledge
2 Park Square, Milton Park, Abingdon, Oxon OX14 4RN

Simultaneously published in the USA and Canada
by Routledge
711 Third Avenue, New York, NY 10017

Routledge is an imprint of the Taylor & Francis Group, an informa business

British Library Cataloguing in Publication Data
A catalogue record for this book is available from the British Library

Library of Congress Cataloging in Publication Data
Jones, Rodney H.
Health and Risk Communication : An Applied Linguistic
Perspective / Rodney H. Jones.
pages cm
Includes bibliographical references and index.
1. Communication in medicine. 2. Physician and patient.
3. Applied linguistics. I. Title.
R118.J66 2013
610 – dc23
2012042956

ISBN: 978-0-415-67259-7 (hbk)
ISBN: 978-0-415-67260-3 (pbk)
ISBN: 978-0-203-52141-0 (ebk)

Typeset in Bembo
by Taylor & Francis Books

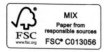

Printed and bound in Great Britain by
TJ International Ltd, Padstow, Cornwall

For my parents

CONTENTS

LIST OF ILLUSTRATIONS

Figures

ACKNOWLEDGEMENTS

So many individuals and organizations have assisted in the research that made this book possible that it would be impossible to mention them all. I am particularly indebted to the staff and volunteers of AIDS Concern (Hong Kong), The Warehouse, and Operation Dawn, as well as various doctors and patients at Queen Elizabeth Hospital. Some of the work reported here was made possible by grants from the Health Care and Promotion Fund (Grant # 257102), the AIDS Trust Fund (Grant # PPE227), and the Hong Kong Research Grants Council General Research Fund (Grant # CityU 144110). Special thanks also go to my mentors and colleagues, especially Ron and Suzanne Scollon, and Chris and Sally Candlin, who have provided guidance and inspiration over the years. Finally, I would like to thank Danyal Freeman for his valuable comments and editorial support and Lynn Zhang and Li Chi Hang for assistance in preparing the bibliography and index. As usual, while I am indebted to these individuals and organizations for their help and support, any inaccuracies or omissions in this manuscript are my responsibility alone.

The author and publishers would like to thank the following copyright holders for permission to reproduce the following material:

Extract from BBC Horizon episode "Does the MMR Jab Cause Autism?" reproduced with kind permission of the BBC Commercial Agency (Chapter 3).

Figure 3.1 'Measles', from *MMR: The Facts* (NHS, 2004), reproduced under Crown Copyright.

Figure 5.1 'Burke's pentad of motives', adapted from R. Scollon and S. W. Scollon, *Nexus analysis: Discourse and the emerging internet* (London: Routledge, 2004), p. 127. Reproduced with kind permission from Routledge.

Figure 5.2 'Constructing risk across timescales and trajectories: Gay men's stories of sexual encounters' from R. H. Jones and C. N. Candlin, *Health, Risk and Society* (London: Routledge, 2003), p. 206. Reproduced with kind permission from Routledge.

Figure 6.1 'Biohazard tattoo' from istolethetv, available for use under the Creative Commons license.

Extract 'A Story of Misdiagnosis: How a wrong diagnosis became a source of motivation', © 2012 Trisha Torrey (http://patients.about.com). Used with permission of About Inc., which can be found online at www.about.com. All rights reserved (Chapter 6).

While the author and publishers have made every effort to contact copyright holders of material used in this volume, they would be grateful to hear from any they were unable to contact.

TRANSCRIPTION CONVENTIONS

=	latching
[	overlapping speech
^	rising intonation
(.)	a pause of less than two tenths of a second
(.3)	number in brackets indicates length of pause
:	drawn-out vowel sound
(word)	inaudible or best guess
((laughter))	non-verbal behavior

The original transcriptions of the examples used from previously published research may employ different transcription conventions. For the purpose of uniformity, all transcriptions have been adapted to conform to the above conventions.

1

COMMUNICATING HEALTH AND RISK

'The thing I'm most worried about,' I told my sisters over Christmas dinner, 'is Alzheimer's. Because there's nothing you can do about it.'

We're debating the pros and cons of my decision to have my genome analysed by a company in California called 23andMe. All you have to do is spit into a test tube and six weeks later they report back to you through a secure website about your ancestry, your susceptibility to a host of diseases, and the presence of genetic markers for various traits like physical endurance and whether or not your urine smells funny after eating asparagus. The company also provides a social networking platform through which customers can share their genetic information with one another and participate in scientific research.

I explain to my sisters how the test will help me to make better health decisions. I'll find out, for example, how often I should have a colonoscopy or a test for glaucoma and whether or not I should keep eating meat or return to the vegetarian diet I maintained in my youth. There is also, I have to admit, a certain prurient curiosity on my part at the prospect of peeking into the 'secret' of my own genetic code. But my sisters are skeptical. And they are not alone. Many experts have grave misgivings about such services, arguing that laypeople don't have sufficient knowledge to interpret genetic data. They also point out that while some knowledge is 'actionable' – if you find you are susceptible to heart disease, for example, you can adjust your diet or your exercise regimen – there is nothing you can do about other kinds of knowledge – except worry. The presence of a variant of the APOE gene associated with Alzheimer's disease is an example. In fact, when the famous geneticist James Watson had his genome scanned, he explicitly instructed scientists to leave information on the APOE gene out of his report.

I'm discussing this with my sisters because I need to know how much they want me to tell them about my results, since whatever I find out about my 'genetic fate' will also likely apply to them. My younger sister cautiously agrees to be privy to my report. My older sister, on the other hand, wants nothing to do with it.

'I don't want to know,' she says. 'Too much knowledge is a dangerous thing'.

*

On September 18, 2007, one day after her book *Louder than Words: A Mother's Journey in Healing Autism* was released, actress Jenny McCarthy appeared on *The Oprah Winfrey Show* to talk about how she came to believe that vaccinations had caused her son's autism and that he could be cured with a special diet free of wheat and dairy products.

She said that the first thing she did after she received her son's diagnosis was to type the word 'autism' into Google. To her surprise, one of the first websites to be returned by her search claimed that autism was reversible and treatable. At first she didn't believe it. She figured that if autism were really reversible and treatable, she would have seen it on *Oprah*. But the more she read, the more convinced she became.

When asked by Oprah how she decided which of the things she read on the internet were true and which weren't, McCarthy summed up her decision-making process with two words: 'Mommy instinct'.

*

At a public forum entitled 'Speaking about Sex in Silent Spaces' held at the University of California at Berkeley in 1999, a middle-aged man stood up and relayed the following story to a hushed crowd:

> So it was a weird thing, we're using a condom but we're talking about 'yeah, I'm going to come inside you and I'm gonna fuck you without a condom,' that sort of thing. And it was just really hot and very compelling ... and we pull off the condom, and we're doing it.
>
> And you know I'm not high, I'm on no drugs. I am who I am. I know what's going on, and it's really hot, it's really compelling. He comes inside me, it's really brief, he pulls out. I get off and I'm nearly in tears now, it's all hitting me like, 'How could I do this, what did I just do, oh my God. I just broke this intense barrier. I went on the other side.'
>
> *(Cotten et al., 1999)*

The year 1999 marked the beginning of a resurgence of HIV infection among gay men in industrialized countries after rates of transmission had been on the decline for more than a decade. Between 2000 and 2005, new HIV diagnoses among men who have sex with men in the United States rose by more than 13 percent (Centers for Disease Control and Prevention, 2007), and in Europe they increased by almost 55 percent (Herida et al., 2007). Against the backdrop of declining HIV prevalence among other groups, the group that in many countries has the most access to information about how to prevent infection continues to be disproportionately affected by the virus. There are many possible explanations for this: a feeling that, because of effective anti-retroviral treatments, HIV infection is not so bad, the popularity of drugs like methamphetamines and ecstasy that affect people's sexual decision-making, and, of course, the internet, which makes hooking up for casual sex easier than ever before. None of these explanations, however, can fully account for what happened to the man who told the story above. None of the conventional explanations are able to penetrate that moment when the words this man and his partner were speaking were suddenly transformed into actions, when they 'went to the other side'.

*

The theme of this book is the relationship between *discourse* – what we say, write, and otherwise communicate about health and risk – and *action* – what we actually do in our everyday lives that affects our health. What these three stories dramatically illustrate is the fact that this relationship is not simple or straightforward. Our response to health-related discourse is not always predictable. Sometimes we neglect easily perceptible risks, and amplify 'virtual' ones, we give credence to the opinions expressed on internet websites and ignore the assessments of experts, and we even appropriate the language of health and safety in ways that may facilitate unsafe or unhealthy behaviors. These stories show how in communicating about health and risk people draw from a wide range of different sources as diverse as biomedical discourse, television talk shows, and their own sexual fantasies. They also demonstrate that many of the most important conversations that people have around health do not occur in clinics or hospitals, but rather in other places like bedrooms and around dinner tables, and the people who most influence our health may not be our doctors, but rather our sexual partners, our friends, our family members, or our favorite television personalities.

Talking about health in any context is a complicated thing, first because when one is talking about health one is usually talking about other things as well, things like fear, trust, commitment, love, money, morality, politics and death, just to name a few. Second, communicating about health can be used to accomplish many different social actions from making an insurance claim, to making love, to making conversation around the dinner table, and how one talks about it depends on what one is doing with the talk.

It is the aim of this book to show how applied linguistics provides uniquely effective tools with which to understand the complex relationship between how people communicate and the actions that they perform around health and risk, actions like having a genetic test, putting on a condom before sex, and taking a child to be immunized against measles. I will describe the ways applied linguistics can deepen our understanding of how people make sense of and use medical and media texts such as health promotion pamphlets and pharmaceutical advertisements, as well as how they conduct interactions around health and risk both with professionals like doctors and nurses, and with other people like friends and family members.

Health and risk in the twenty-first century

Although the main aim of this book is to review the kinds of contributions applied linguistics can make to our understanding of health and risk, an equally important aim is to demonstrate how attention to health and risk can challenge applied linguists to more fully engage with a number of fundamental issues associated with communication in post-modern societies: issues arising from the changing nature of expertise and authority, the erosion of traditional social, disciplinary and institutional boundaries in many domains of life, and the increasing role of technology in mediating our experiences.

The multiple ways in which health and risk are constructed in contemporary societies are complex and paradoxical. At no time in history have humans enjoyed longer lives and better health and had access to such sophisticated tools for assessing and addressing health risks. At the same time, these incredible advances in biomedicine and public health seem to have engendered among many people more rather than less anxiety about their health as they find themselves having to negotiate an increasingly voluminous and contradictory array of health-related discourses. In the 1980s the cultural critic Paula Treichler (1988b) used the term 'epidemic of significance' to refer to the discursive environment surrounding AIDS. Today this term seems an apt description of the discursive environment around health in general. Discourse about health and risk has reached 'epidemic proportions'.

What is 'health'?

One major reason for the proliferation of discourse about health and risk has been the shift in industrialized countries from a preoccupation with communicable diseases like tuberculosis and polio, to a focus on chronic conditions like heart disease, cancer, and other illnesses related to lifestyle and behavior, primarily thanks to advances in antimicrobials and hygiene throughout the twentieth century (Institute for the Future, 2003; Lalonde, 1974). What this has meant is that, at least in richer societies, illness has come to be seen less as a result of external risks and more as a result of individual behavior. The focus of health-related discourse has moved away from the curing of illness to the maintenance of health.

There has also been a discursive 'upping of the ante' in the way we define health. No longer is it just a matter of being free from disease. It is now, according to the World Health Organization's 1978 Alma Ata Declaration, something much more ambitious: 'a state of complete physical, mental and social well-being'. While this redefinition is useful in highlighting the important psychological and social dimensions of health, it is hard to imagine many people who would describe themselves as being in this state. Instead, the 'worried well' of the developed world find themselves spending more and more time and money in search of a seemingly unattainable state of 'wellness', a state which they are meant to display to others through a combination of ways of speaking, and behaviors around diet, exercise, fashion, and drug and alcohol consumption (Davison and Smith, 1995; Skrabanek, 1994). In other words, health has become not just a matter of physical, mental and social well-being, but primarily a *discursive* exercise of constantly reproducing 'health' in our daily lives as part of ongoing identity projects (Giddens, 1991; Kellner, 1992). The consequence of this has been the increasing 'medicalization' of everyday life in which nearly every moment is the potential site of a 'health decision', whether it has to do with where we live, what we eat, who we have sex with, or what kinds of consumer products we buy (Lupton, 1995; Prior, 2000).

At the same time, the access laypeople have to knowledge about health and risk is also changing. No longer solely the property of experts, medical information circulates freely through the print and electronic media, public discourse, and the everyday conversations of laypeople, being constantly reinterpreted and repackaged as it moves from scientific journals to newspaper reports to online social networking sites to dinner-table conversations. On the one hand, greater and greater hopes are pinned on biomedical advances as the solution to all of our woes, while on the other hand, people are increasingly skeptical of biomedical discourse, which seems every day to yield a different set of pronouncements about what's 'good for us' and what's not. The more we are able to calculate and 'manage' our health risks, the more uncertain and unpredictable our lives seem to become (Beck, 1992).

The new ways health and illness are coming to be defined and represented in discourse present a number of challenging questions for applied linguists: questions about the ways social practices and social identities are constructed, maintained, promoted and undermined in texts about health, questions about how meanings associated with health and risk change as they travel from genre to genre and context to context, and questions about how particular discursive constructions of health and illness create affordances and constraints on how people can think about their health and what they can do about it.

Interacting around health and risk

Along with these changing discursive constructions of health and risk in public discourse have also come dramatic changes in the 'interaction orders' (Goffman, 1983) within which people negotiate health risks and exchange health-related goods and services. Since the 1950s expectations about how health professionals and their clients are supposed to treat each other have undergone a profound trans-formation. The most prominent aspect of this has been a move away from expecta-tions that patients comply unquestioningly with doctors' instructions towards models in which medical consultations are seen as exercises in 'shared decision-making'.

Much of the impetus for this change came out of a realization within the medical establishment itself in the 1970s and 1980s that more patient participation in care resulted in better health outcomes (Katz, 1984; Korsch and Negrete, 1972). Since the mid-1980s, 'effective communication' has regularly been championed in the medical literature as an essential aspect of effective clinical care (Armstrong, 1984; Lupton, 2003).

At the same time, with the increasing fragmentation and specialization of health services, the number of different kinds of professionals people interact with around their health has increased, and these different professionals often speak 'different languages' and structure interactions with clients differently. Furthermore, within institutions, healthcare workers from different disciplines are increasingly required to interact in teams in which they must be accountable not just for their professional differences but also for their different ways of communicating (Iedema, 2003a; Iedema and Scheeres, 2003). People also regularly engage in conversations about health with people outside of mainstream medical professions, like massage therapists, yoga teachers and health food store clerks, not to mention financial advisers and the representatives of insurance companies. Finally, with the heightened awareness of health and risk in everyday life, more and more of our daily interactions around activities like eating, sex, shopping, parenting, work and recreation have become occasions for conversations about health and risk.

These new orders of interaction around health and risk also present a number of challenging questions for applied linguists, questions about what constitutes 'effective communication' in healthcare encounters and whose agenda it is designed to promote, questions about how people in various settings enact and negotiate power and expertise around questions of health and risk, and questions about the new kinds of discursive demands that are being made on people both inside and outside of institutional settings in encounters having to do with health (Sarangi and Roberts, 1999).

Technology and the body

Yet another important change in the way we communicate about health and risk has to do with the fact that, more and more, our experiences of our bodies are mediated through technologies of representation like laboratory tests and high-tech scans. One consequence of this is that the body as an object of medical knowledge has become increasingly separated from the actual physical body of the patient (Atkinson, 1995; Berg and Bowker, 1997; Iedema, 2003b). Doctors spend less time examining their patients' bodies, and more time examining texts about these bodies, to the point where some fear that the ability to make an accurate diagnosis using a physical examination is a dying art (Sanders, 1956). The decrease in human contact between doctors and patients is only likely to increase with the use of remote monitoring devices, which make clinic visits less necessary (Topol, 2012).

This increased entextualization of the body is not just occurring in institutional contexts. People themselves now have access to tools with which to monitor and record their own bodily functions and to share this data with other people via the internet, as well as access to high-tech medical testing services in areas like genetics, pregnancy, and HIV infection, which in the past were only available to physicians (Fernandez-Luke et al., 2009; Goetz, 2010; Sarasohn-Kahn, 2008).

These new technologies of representation used in discourse about health and risk also present applied linguists with a number of important questions, questions about who has access to different kinds of resources for entextualizing the body, about who ultimately 'owns' or controls these representations, and about the different kinds of social actions and social identities that are made possible or constrained by them.

Cultures, communities, and social networks

Finally, communication about health and risk is performed within progressively more complex webs of social relationships. Healthcare settings are becoming increasingly 'multicultural', with patients coming from a variety of different backgrounds and healthcare workers finding themselves working across cultural and professional boundaries. These settings have also become increasingly bureaucratic (Strong, 2001), with physicians, nurses, and patients having to render themselves accountable to a greater range of people.

Outside of institutions, health and risk-related communication takes place within a multiplicity of other groups: peer groups, support groups, 'communities', and social networks. Sometimes the main purpose of talk about health and risk, in fact, is to claim for oneself or impute to others membership in some social group. Epidemiologists and public health workers impute to people membership in 'risk groups'. People suffering from various ailments build communities and support groups based on their shared experiences of suffering or discrimination. And even people who share risk behaviors bond together and cultivate a sense of common identity. With the advent of the internet, new forms of social organization, such as online communities and social networks, with their own unique forms of discourse, are changing the way information about health and risk circulates and the possibilities open to individuals for managing both their health and their social identities.

The questions these various forms of social organization present to applied linguists include those about the role discourse plays in constructing 'cultures', communities, institutions, and social networks, questions about how people manage their membership in multiple overlapping and intersecting social groups, and questions about how interactions around health and risk are used strategically to claim and impute membership in these groups.

The organization of this book

This book is organized around the four challenges that health and risk communication presents to applied linguistics that I outlined above. After a discussion of the theoretical perspective and analytical tools of an applied linguistic approach in this chapter and the next, I will explore in chapter 3 how texts like scientific papers, newspaper articles, health promotion pamphlets, and drug labels function to construct particular 'versions of reality' around health and risk, and the ways health-related meanings change as they move across these genres.

In chapters 4 and 5 I will move on to examine different situated encounters, from medical consultations to dinner table conversations, in which people talk about and take actions related to health and risk. Chapter 4 will focus on professional encounters in clinics and hospitals, exploring how various kinds of healthcare workers such as doctors, nurses, and genetic counselors negotiate issues of power and expertise with patients. In chapter 5 I will focus on interactions outside of institutional settings, exploring how people negotiate health and risk in their everyday lives with friends, family members, and sexual partners.

In chapters 6 and 7 I will analyze the various ways in which the body itself is transformed into a text in the context of health and risk communication. In chapter 6 I will focus on more traditional ways of entextualizing the body in medicine, namely diagnosis and narrative, and in chapter 7 I will focus on more recent trends in high-tech entextualization and the challenges these present to patients, healthcare professionals, and analysts.

In chapter 8 I will discuss the roles various social groups such as 'cultures', communities, and social networks play in communication around health and risk, and the role discourse plays in the formation and maintenance of these groups. I will also consider new forms of social organization such as online communities and social networks and examine how patterns of communication within these groups affect the ways knowledge about health and risk is created and used.

The final chapter will present an overview of the concepts I have discussed throughout the book, as well as a discussion of the practical implications of applied linguistic research in health and risk communication.

Intellectual roots of an applied linguistic approach

An applied linguistic approach to health and risk integrates concepts and methods from linguistics with those from many other disciplines, particularly sociology, anthropology, and cultural studies. Work in these other disciplines has not just helped to lay the intellectual foundations for the applied linguistic approach to health and risk communication I will develop in this book. It has also set the parameters for a number of broader academic debates which will arise as recurring themes in the chapters that follow: the debate between micro-analytical approaches which focus on the fine-grained aspects of social interaction and more macro-analytical approaches which examine broader social formations; the debate over the extent to which individuals can exert agency when it comes to health-related behavior and the extent to which they are constrained and governed by social structures; and the debate about the role of social scientists *vis-à-vis* the biomedical establishment: whether scholars should engage in a social science *for* medicine, which seeks to contribute to developing and refining the disciplinary techniques of biomedicine and health promotion, or a social science *of* medicine, which seeks to problematize and, in some cases, disrupt those techniques (Nettleton and Bunton, 1995; Straus, 1957).

Although social scientists and humanities scholars often complain about playing second fiddle to scientists in discussions of health and risk, the last half-century has seen a significant shift in health-related fields from a focus on 'technological' solutions alone to one which recognizes the importance of the 'social' aspects of health. Moreover, this shift has come at a time when many social sciences themselves have been experiencing a 'discursive turn', a greater appreciation of the role of language and other semiotic systems in constituting social realities (Harré, 2003; Jaworski and Coupland, 1999).

Eliot Mishler and the 'voices' of the medical encounter

Among the most influential figures in applied linguistic approaches to health and risk communication is the social psychologist Eliot Mishler (1984; Mishler et al., 1981), whose classic observation that medical encounters often involve a 'struggle' between the competing 'voices' of the patient's lifeworld and of the world of medicine serves as the starting point for many investigations of clinical communication. Mishler's observation came from the extensive analysis of tape-recorded medical interviews in which he shows that doctors and patients continually vie to have their voices heard, with the technical rationalism of the doctor more often than not winning out against the more socially oriented and intuitive voice of the patient. Others have extended this idea to contexts outside of consultations, with Atkinson (1995), for example, arguing that the interaction between these competing voices is also characteristic of physician–physician discourse.

What Mishler means by 'voices', of course, goes well beyond what individual doctors or individual patients say during a consultation. For him, 'a "voice" represents a normative order' (Mishler, 1990, p. 297), a way not just of speaking but also of viewing life, of organizing knowledge, and of relating to other people. In this respect voices are similar to what Gee (2011) would call 'Discourses' (with a capital D), which he defines as:

> ways of combining and integrating language, actions, interactions, ways of thinking, believing, valuing, and using various symbols, tools, and objects to enact a particular sort of socially recognizable identity.
>
> *(p. 201)*

Mishler's observation that the power and authority of doctors comes not just from who they are or what they know, but from how they *talk* opened up a whole new way of thinking about health-related encounters. I begin with Mishler's insight not just because of the overwhelming influence of his work on applied linguistic approaches to health and risk, but also because of the problem he has defined for researchers of understanding just how the concrete situated voice of the speaker and the abstract voice of the 'worldview' through which he or she is speaking are related. What does it mean to speak in the 'voice of medicine', and how can we tell when somebody is doing so? I also choose to start with this idea of competing voices because nowadays the situation has become much more complicated than when Mishler first made his observations in the early 1980s. With increased dissemination of medical knowledge and a blurring of the boundaries between professional and lay expertise, it is sometimes difficult to predict who will speak with the 'voice of medicine' in a clinical encounter: the doctor or the patient (Sarangi and Clarke, 2002).

Narratives of health and illness

Another area of health and risk communication where social scientists have done considerable work is in the analysis of illness narratives. Scholars of narrative in sociology (see for example Frank, 1995; Hydén, 1997; Mishler, 1986), as well as in anthropology (see for example Garro, 1994; Good, 1994; Kleinman, 1986; Mattingly and Garro, 2000), have explored how people use stories to organize and 'make sense' (Bruner, 1985) of their illnesses by fitting them into culturally recognizable and acceptable patterns. Some, such as Kleinman (1986), go so far as to insist that narratives are not just reflections of the illness experience, but also contribute to *creating* that experience as it is lived by individuals. On a practical level, interest in narrative from social scientists has led to a movement within medicine itself to pay more attention to patients' narratives as a way of improving clinical care (see for example Charon, 2001; Greenhalgh and Hurwitz, 1998).

This interest in narrative, particularly its attention to the ways in which discourse organizes reality, is, of course, naturally attractive to applied linguists. At the same time, research on narrative and illness in medical sociology and anthropology has also been criticized for not paying sufficient attention to the ways narratives are affected by the social contexts in which they are told (Atkinson, 1997; Atkinson and Silverman, 1997; Sandelowski, 2002). An applied linguistic approach to health and risk is concerned not just with the contents of people's narratives, but also in the ways they are socially occasioned and embedded into different social contexts (see chapter 6).

Identity

Another way in which sociology has influenced applied linguistic approaches to health and risk concerns its insights into the issue of social identity. Early work in medical sociology concentrated on the various 'roles' societies make available for people to adopt in their interactions around health and illness. The most famous treatment of this type is Parsons' (1951) description of the 'sick role', a set of norms and expectations in contemporary western societies which places certain demands upon the sick person while at the same time exempting him or her from certain social obligations. More recently, sociologists have focused on the changing nature of the sick role as medicine becomes more market oriented and the sick come to be treated as 'customers' (see for example Henderson, 2002).

Of more interest to applied linguists, however, is work which helps to reveal the ways such roles as 'doctor' and 'patient' are *dynamically* constructed and *strategically* performed. The scholar who is of most interest in this regard, of course, is Erving Goffman. Not only does Goffman's body of work contain research directly focusing on medical institutions (1961) and the ways people with outward manifestations of illness manage their identities (1963), but his dramaturgical approach to social interaction (1959) has influenced a host of studies in the sociology of medicine. Linguists, especially those working in the tradition of interactional sociolinguistics (see for example J. Coupland, Robinson, and Coupland, 1994; Hamilton, 2003, 2004; Myers, 2003; C. Roberts, Sarangi and Moss, 2004; F. D. Roberts, 1999; Sarangi and Roberts, 1999; Tannen and Wallat, 1987), owe a particular debt to Goffman for the practical analytical tools that he has provided to them, particularly the concepts of 'face' (1959) and 'framing' (1974) (see chapter 4).

The organization of everyday life

The branch of sociology that has arguably had the most profound influence on applied linguistics and the way it approaches health and risk communication is ethnomethodology. Developed by American sociologist Harold Garfinkel (1967), ethnomethodology focuses on everyday activities as methods through which people make sense of the social world and make themselves 'accountable' to one another. From the beginning, ethnomethodologists have taken a particular interest in medical and therapeutic encounters. In fact, nearly half of the papers in Garfinkel's landmark *Studies in Ethnomethodology* (1967) deal with interaction in healthcare settings of some kind, and David Sudnow's *Passing On: The Social Organization of Dying* (1967), published in the same year, can be regarded as the first book-length study in medical ethnomethodology (ten Have, 1995). Even the early work by Sacks (1967, 1972) in conversation analysis, the outgrowth of ethnomethodology that has most strongly impacted applied linguistics, focused on contexts in which issues of health and risk are strongly implicated: suicide hotlines and group therapy sessions.

The chief contribution of ethnomethodology to studies of health and risk is its attention to how social identities like 'doctor' and 'patient' as well as other 'social facts' like 'illness' and 'risk' are constituted moment by moment as people engage in their daily routinized encounters with one another. In contrast, then, to Parsons' view of the 'sick role' as a static set of rights and responsibilities granted by society, and even to Goffman's view of the sick role as a matter of strategic performance, ethnomethodology sees the sick role as something that is organizationally realized through the repetitive performance of various social and professional practices, many of them rather banal in nature.

This perspective, as I said above, has been enormously influential in applied linguistics, and the 1980s and 1990s saw a proliferation of ethnomethodology-inspired studies of physician–patient interaction, some of which I will review in chapter 4. Ethnomethodological approaches and the fine-grained conversation analytical studies that grew out of them have, however, also attracted criticism from those who find the method's reluctance to look beyond the narrow confines of the interaction itself too limiting (see for example Lynch and Bogen, 1994). While their focus on the micro-politics of interaction can reveal much, for example, about how doctors maintain power over patients on the level of the medical encounter, studies inspired by ethnomethodology are less able to link this to broader workings of power on the level of institutions, societies, and cultures. They also tend to be less sensitive to the ways particular encounters are embedded within wider arrangements of medical work, institutional systems and policies that may have a profound effect on participants even when they do not explicitly orient towards them (Pappas, 1990).

Social contexts and culture

In contrast to the micro-analytical perspective of ethnomethodology is the work of medical anthropologists, who focus on how culture affects our experiences of health and risk. Medical anthropology's attention to cultural models and group processes has acted as a strong counterweight to the overwhelming 'methodological individualism' (Udéhn, 2001) of many approaches to health communication, as well as to the preoccupation of micro-analytical approaches such as ethnomethodology with the fine details of situated talk.

Medical anthropologists have attempted to understand local meanings and 'folk' models of health, illness and risk by, for example, describing various systems of classification of diseases and 'dangers' (Young and Garro, 1993). Particularly significant in this regard has been the work of Mary Douglas, whose research on cultural constructions of hygiene (1966) highlights how talk about health and risk is inextricably intertwined with issues of social order and control. Also influential is the work of Arthur Kleinman (1986), a psychiatrist and anthropologist, whose research on mental illness in China has contributed to our understanding of how people's 'explanatory models' of illness can vary widely across cultures.

Perhaps the most important contribution anthropology has made to applied linguistic approaches to health and risk is methodological rather than theoretical. While in the 1980s and 1990s studies relying solely on conversation analytical tools tended to dominate, today many applied linguists interested in health and risk are coming to embrace more ethnographic approaches which involve such methods as in-depth interviewing and participant observation as a way to supplement the close analysis of texts and conversational transcripts (see for example Ainsworth-Vaughn, 1998; Coupland et al., 1991; Gwyn, 2002; Sarangi and Roberts, 1999; Slade et al., 2008). Among the most cogent and oft-quoted proponents of this approach is Cicourel (1992), whose persuasive demonstration of how, without reference to larger aspects of context, many transcriptions of medical encounters are difficult to make sense of led him to call for increased 'ecological validity' in discourse analytical studies of medical encounters.

Knowledge and power

The final set of contributions to applied linguistic approaches to health and risk that bear mentioning comes from the field of cultural studies, especially as it has been influenced by the work of the French philosopher Michel Foucault, who, in a number of landmark works including *Madness and Civilization* (1967), *The Birth of the Clinic* (1976) and the three volumes of *The History of Sexuality* (1978–88) argues that biomedical knowledge, and indeed all 'knowledge', is part of the 'disciplinary apparatus' of society. Power, according to Foucault, comes not from force or coercion, but from the construction of knowledge through 'orders of discourse', which delineate and constrain what people can do, say and even think when it comes to things like health, illness, deviance, and risk. These orders of discourse are continually reproduced not just in institutional encounters like medical consultations, but also through education, commercial advertising, the media, entertainment and popular culture (Armstrong, 1983).

Cultural critics in the Foucaultian mold have studied myriad aspects of health and risk from the cultural construction of 'new' diseases like chronic fatigue syndrome, depression, and attention deficit disorder (Morris, 1998) to patterns of consumption around 'body maintenance' such as diets and fitness centers (see for example Featherstone, 1991; Turner, 1992). This perspective was particularly influential in the early days of the AIDS epidemic, with the work of critics like Paula Treichler (1988a, 1988b), Simon Watney (1989, 1990, 1993), and Cindy Patton (1990). AIDS gave scholars in the field of cultural studies the opportunity to observe first-hand the ways discourses around disease, even the purportedly 'objective' discourse of biomedicine, promote particular ideologies and social structures. While Mishler pointed to the dominance of the 'voice of medicine' in institutional interactions around health, and ethnomethodologists showed how that dominance is inter-actionally accomplished, those working in the field of cultural studies have endeavored to show how such dominance operates on the broader level through the discursive construction of bodies of knowledge that legitimate certain social practices and social identities and marginalize others.

The major contribution of such studies to applied linguistic perspectives on health and risk is the theoretical construct of the 'order of discourse', a construct which re-emerges in several schools of linguistic discourse analysis, in particular, critical discourse analysis (Fairclough, 1992a, 1992b), new literacy studies (Gee, 2011) and mediated discourse analysis (Scollon, 2001b; Scollon et al., 2012). For Foucault and those who took up this idea after him, orders of discourse are ways of speaking about certain topics that promote certain kinds of values, social relationships, and 'versions of reality'. He gives as examples 'clinical discourse, economic discourse, the discourse of natural history, [and] psychiatric discourse' (Foucault, 1972, p. 121). Orders of discourse (or, as I will be calling them, 'discourses') can in some respects be seen as the repositories of the 'voices' of which Mishler speaks. The 'voice of medicine' that governs the interaction between a doctor and a patient is the instantiation of a broader 'discourse of medicine' which supports and maintains the practices and social identities of institutions like clinics, hospitals, public health services, and medical schools.

Another important contribution of this approach, and one closely related to the notion of orders of discourse, is the concept of intertextuality (Kristeva, 1980), the idea that all texts and utterances are linked in complex ways with other texts and utterances, ways which sometimes combine or play the voices of different discourses off of each other. Communication around health and risk never involves a single, unitary voice, or even just the two voices identified by Mishler, but rather it forms, in Treichler's (1988b, p. 42) words, a 'nexus where multiple meanings, stories and discourses intersect and overlap, reinforce and subvert one another.' Medical voices compete not just with the voice of the 'lifeworld', but also with religious voices, commercial voices, political voices, and the voices of multiple professions, communities and interest groups. In order to understand this chorus of voices, Treichler (1988b, p. 68) argues, 'we need an epidemiology of signification, a comprehensive mapping and analysis of these multiple meanings.'

The degree to which cultural studies provides the tools to conduct such an 'epidemiology of signification', however, is unclear, for to do so requires some attention to the actual linguistic mechanisms through which knowledge is constructed and power is exercised on the level of concrete texts and situated utterances. Some have criticized cultural studies for what they see as a preference for theorizing at the broader level of 'discourses' to examining how these 'discourses' are actually instantiated in the 'nuts and bolts' of texts and talk. Lemke (1995, p. 29), for example, complains that:

> It is not possible to know in terms of linguistic features of texts exactly how to interpret many of Foucault's theoretical principles, and while he sketches the general principles, there are no specific examples to show us actually how to analyze the relations of specific texts.

*

Although the applied linguistic approach to health and risk communication I will outline in this book draws on concepts from all of these approaches and focuses on many of the same themes, it differs in significant ways from all of them. One of these ways is in the potential it offers to bridge the 'macro–micro division' (Layder, 1993, p. 102) that separates perspectives like ethnomethodology and microsociology from anthropology and cultural studies by providing a set of tools that allows analysts to understand how broader 'voices' and 'discourses' in texts and talk are constructed at the level of discrete linguistic features and the micro-mechanics of social interaction. Another is in the potential it offers to bridge the gap between discourse and social practice, to understand how things like social roles, systems of classification, ideologies and bodies of 'knowledge' actually affect the concrete social actions that people take around health and risk in their day-to-day lives. In the following chapter I will begin to sketch out the principles of this approach.

2

APPLIED LINGUISTICS

Discourse in action

When I buy a box of Extra Strength Tylenol at the San Francisco airport I'm not just buying relief from my chronic back pain. I'm also buying a 'text' in the form of the package that the product comes in. The front of the package, with its familiar white lettering against a red background, identifies the product as a 'pain reliever' and 'fever reducer', and informs me that it comes in the form of 'easy to swallow EZ TABS', two of which are pictured on the package with rays of light emanating from them like Underdog's 'super energy pill' from the cartoons I watched as a child. The words on the side of the package address me directly:

> Think about this: The pure pain relief in TYLENOL® works fast on your headache and won't irritate your stomach lining the way that aspirin, naproxen sodium, or even ibuprofen can.
>
> TYLENOL® is considered a pain reliever of choice by doctors and leading professional healthcare organizations. When used as directed, TYLENOL® has a superior safety profile compared with other over-the-counter pain relievers.

In two short paragraphs I am introduced to a world of doctors and healthcare organizations, who, fortuitously, have made the same choice of pain relievers as I have. I am also introduced to a world of risk and 'safety profiles'. I am not entirely sure what a 'safety profile' is, but the characterization of this product's profile as 'superior' is reassuring. I am introduced to a world of 'other' pain relievers: aspirin, naproxen sodium, and 'even ibuprofen'. I wonder if this business about safety has anything to do with stomach irritation. I briefly wonder why the word 'even' is used with ibuprofen. What's so special about ibuprofen? Finally, I am introduced to two distinct 'voices'. The friendly, intimate voice of the first paragraph which addresses me as 'you' and worries about my stomach being irritated, and the more distant voice of the second paragraph, which uses passive constructions and 'fancy' words like 'leading', 'superior' and 'safety' profile.

When I turn to the back of the package, the whole business about 'safety' comes up again, this time transformed into a specific set of warnings, and the voice once again changes abruptly, this time becoming the voice of an authority figure peppering me with imperatives:

> * Alcohol Warning: If you consume 3 or more alcoholic drinks every day, ask your doctor whether you should take acetaminophen or other pain relievers/fever reducers. Acetaminophen may cause liver damage. Do not use with any other product containing acet-aminophen. Stop use and ask a doctor if new symptoms occur; redness or swelling is present; pain gets worse or lasts for more than 10 days; fever gets worse or lasts for more than 3 days. If pregnant or breast-feeding, ask a health professional before use. Keep out of reach of children. Overdose Warning: Taking more than the recommended dose (overdose) may cause liver damage. In case of overdose, get medical help or contact a Poison Control Center right away. Quick medical attention is critical for adults as well as for children even if you do not notice any signs or symptoms. Do not use if carton is opened or neck wrap or foil inner seal imprinted with Safety Seal® is broken or missing.

This part of the package also represents a world of healthcare profes-sionals and institutions (doctors, Poison Control Centers) as well as other kinds of people (adults, children, pregnant women) who are placed in certain relationships with one another. In addition, there is also a host of 'invisible' people populating this passage: research scientists who conducted studies on the relationship between acetaminophen and liver damage, legislators who drafted laws requiring manufacturers of over-the-counter medications to include certain information on their packages, lawyers who reviewed this part of the package for the company to make sure it covers them against liability stemming from any consequences (such as liver damage) that might result from the use of this product.

In short, this simple package of Tylenol is a complex chorus of different 'voices': the voices of doctors and biomedical researchers, of advertisers and marketers, of 'product safety' and quality control specialists, and of lawyers and government regulators. Each voice in this chorus links the text to complex chains of discourse and action, some of which I am conscious of, and others which are hidden from me.

The warning not to use if the 'neck wrap or foil inner seal imprinted with Safety Seal® is broken or missing', for instance, links the text to a chain of discourse and action that began back in 1982 when seven people died after taking cyanide-laced Tylenol in the Chicago area, causing a national panic in the United States and a precipitous decline in Tylenol's market share. The 'Safety Seal' technology was part of Johnson and Johnson's effort to restore confidence in the brand, an effort which was so successful that it has come to be regarded as a 'textbook case' in successful crisis management (Berg and Robb, 1992).

The warnings about liver damage link the package to more recent research about the dangers of acetaminophen (the leading cause of acute liver failure in the United States), to newspaper articles reporting this research, to lawsuits, and to public accusations of corporate irresponsibility leveled at the manufacturers by consumer groups. And the directions not to take more than six tablets in 24 hours link the text to a recent decision made by McNeil-PPC (a division of Johnson and Johnson), partly in response to these accusations, to revise its maximum daily dosage, and to the press release announcing this change. In that press release the public is reminded that 'Acetaminophen, the active ingredient in TYLENOL®, ... [is] safe when used as directed ... [and] remains the brand of pain reliever that doctors recommend more than any other and that hospitals use most' (McNeil-PPC, 2011).

*

My musings above about the Tylenol package illustrate the two main issues about language and its relationship to health and risk that are at the center of the applied linguistic approach I will be developing in this book. First, this text, like most texts about health, is *heteroglossic* (Bakhtin, 1981; Gee, 2011). That is, it brings together the 'voices' of many different kinds of people: marketers, medical professionals and government regulators, and the way these voices mix and interact with one another is crucial to how I am able to understand and use this text. Each of these voices represents a particular 'discourse'; each constructs a particular 'version of reality' which includes certain kinds of people and certain kinds of social practices and excludes others; and each creates certain versions of 'me' as a reader, inviting me to assume a number of different identities: the identity of a customer, of a patient, of a parent, of a heavy drinker, and of a pregnant woman. Each of these voices also has a particular *agenda*. Sometimes that agenda is directly related to me (for example, getting me to buy the product), and sometimes it is less related to me personally (for example, complying with government regulations or reducing legal liability). None of these voices, even the apparently 'objective' voice of biomedicine, is ideologically neutral.

Second, this text is linked to many other texts – newspaper stories, research reports, government regulations, conversations with doctors and other healthcare professionals – in multiple chains of *discourse and action*. It is part of a chain of discourse and action, for example, involving me, that began with my injuring my back while trying to lift a heavy case into the overhead bin on a flight from Hong Kong to New York, a chain which extends through visits to various professionals – a physician, a radiologist, a physiotherapist, an acupuncturist – to the moment when, before taking another long-haul flight I bought this package of Tylenol in an airport shop. It is also part of a chain of discourse and action involving the manufacturer, a chain which extends many years back, even before the infamous poisonings of 1982, and includes thousands of corporate meetings, public relations campaigns, private conversations in offices, memos, lawsuits and press releases. What an applied linguistic approach to health and risk communication seeks to understand is how these disparate chains of discourse and action are linked together, and how these linkages affect things like the manufacturer's decision to change its dosage recommendations and my own decision to buy this particular pain reliever.

Applied linguistics

Over the past three decades there has been a surge of interest from applied linguists in communication around health and risk (Brown et al., 2006; Candlin and Candlin, 2003; Sarangi, 2004). While much of this interest has been in physician–patient communication, applied linguists have also focused on the discourse of health promotion texts, the construction of health and risk in the media, the role of technology in interactions around health and risk, and the discursive negotiation of health and risk in everyday life.

What distinguishes an applied linguistic approach to health and risk from those of disciplines like communication studies and medical sociology is its focus on *language in use*, or, to put it another way, 'discourse in action' (Norris and Jones, 2005). Applied linguistics regards language as not just a means for exchanging information but as a means of *performing social actions* – we don't just 'mean' things with words, we 'do things' with them (Austin, 1976); and the fundamental task of applied linguistics is to figure out how people use language and other semiotic systems to perform concrete actions in the world.

I will go even further out on a limb in arguing that *all* social actions depend somewhere along the line on discourse, including apparently solitary or silent actions: even our 'private' thoughts still involve language (what Vygotsky (1987) calls 'inner speech') and even 'private' behavior still involves prior social learning. Discourse is the primary tool we use to act, to interact, and to think. Consequently, it is hard to get a handle on why people act the way they do – whether, for example, they use condoms in casual sexual encounters, take vitamin supplements, apply sunscreen, or take their children to be vaccinated – without understanding how discourse mediates these actions, and how it makes some actions easier and others more difficult. Applied linguistics, with its rich and varied arsenal of analytical tools, provides the resources to help us understand not just how people make meanings around health and risk, but also 'how people "do" health through daily embodied and discursive practice' (Paugh and Izquierdo, 2009, p. 188).

This preoccupation with the relationship between discourse and action is at the core of all of the approaches to health and risk communication I will discuss in this book. Not all of these approaches, however, conceive of this relationship in exactly the same way. Some, like conversation analysis (J. M. Atkinson and Heritage, 1984; H. Sacks, 1972; H. Sacks et al., 1974), view it from a micro-analytical perspective, focusing on the moment-by-moment actions people accomplish in their turns at talk and exploring how events (like visits to the doctor), identities (like 'doctors' and 'patients'), social facts (like 'health' and 'illness'), and even the institutions within which these interactions occur (like hospitals and clinics) are themselves jointly *accomplished* through the moment-by-moment actions of participants. Those taking a more ethnographic approach come at the question of discourse and action from the other direction, beginning with 'macro-analytical' notions like 'community' and 'speech event', and trying to understand the 'competencies' associated with these broader structures and how they govern what people say to each other, where, when and how (Gumperz and Hymes, 1964; Hymes, 1974). Between these two extremes are approaches like pragmatics and interactional sociolinguistics (Levinson, 1979; Schiffrin, 1988; Tannen, 1980, 1982, 1993), which focus on how people negotiate social actions by strategically contextualizing their utterances (Gumperz, 1982) and 'positioning' themselves (Davies and Harré, 1990) in relation to their interlocutors, the topics under discussion, and the social groups they belong to.

The approach to discourse that has particularly influenced the analytical framework I lay out in this book is mediated discourse analysis (Norris and Jones, 2005; Scollon, 2001b), a perspective which focuses on how social actions are *mediated* through discourse and other 'cultural tools' and on how these tools amplify or constrain the kinds of social actions that people can take and the kinds of social identities that they can claim. The main difference between mediated discourse analysis and other approaches to discourse is that rather than beginning with language and other semiotic systems and exploring what kinds of social actions people can take with them, it begins with social actions and asks what role discourse and other cultural tools had in carrying them out. One of the consequences of approaching discourse through action is a realization that we cannot always 'read' social actions off of discourse or expect particular kinds of discourse to be used to perform particular kinds of actions. In my study of discourse about HIV/AIDS in China, for example (Jones, 1999, 2002a, 2002b), I found time and time again that talk about 'safer sex' was often used to perform actions that had very little to do with 'safer sex', and, in fact, was sometimes part of patently unsafe sexual practices. In other words, discourse does not cause actions, and actions do not cause discourse in any direct way. Rather, discourse and action exist in what Wertsch (1994, p. 205) calls a relationship of 'tension between the mediational means as provided in the sociocultural setting and the unique contextualized use of these means in carrying out particular concrete actions'.

Another approach which has influenced my framework is critical discourse analysis (Chouliaraki and Fairclough, 1999; Fairclough, 1992a, 1992b; van Dijk, 1993; Wodak, 1996), an approach which seeks to link lexicogrammatical and interactional features of texts and conversations to the broader systems of knowledge and social practice which Foucault called 'orders of discourse' (or 'discourses'). Unlike those working in the paradigm of cultural studies, critical discourse analysts bring to the study of power and ideology a set of analytical tools which allows them to empirically explore the ways these 'discourses' are actually instantiated in texts and talk.

It is not my aim in this book, however, to argue for the superiority of any particular 'school' of applied linguistics or discourse analysis. Rather, I will present what I believe are the key problems in health and risk communication and explore how a variety of perspectives on *language in use* can be used together to solve them. In fact, it is to a large extent work on health and risk communication that has most dramatically highlighted the necessity of cultivating what Sarangi (2010b, p. 413) calls an 'analytic eclecticism' in applied linguistics. Seeing health and risk communication as a matter of social action means being able to situate it both in the context of the immediate setting with its unique interactional demands and constraints and in the context of the larger socio-cultural environment (Candlin and Candlin, 2003; Cicourel, 1992; Hak, 1999).

'Hearing' voices

And so what can the action-oriented approach to applied linguistics I have been discussing here add to our understanding of health and risk communication? To begin to answer this question I will turn to two fundamental problems in understanding communication that I brought up in the previous chapter. The first is the problem set by Mishler of sorting out the relationship between broader 'ideological voices' (like the 'voice of medicine') and the actual voices of writers and speakers in specific texts and social interactions. How do we know when someone is speaking with the 'voice of medicine' or the 'voice of the lifeworld' or, for that matter, some other 'voice', and what effect does the appropriation of these different voices have on the way we communicate about health and risk? The second is the problem of understanding the relationship between what is said and written about health and risk and what we actually do about it. How do the texts and talk we produce around health and risk actually affect the kinds of actions we can take, and how are these actions transformed by discourse into social practices that are associated with certain kinds of people and the social groups they belong to?

The first problem can be stated succinctly with the question: 'who's speaking here?' The question in part arises from Mishler's (1984, p. 122) classic observation that the medical interview involves the competition of two 'voices': the 'voice of medicine' constructed through 'disinterested observation' and the 'principles of scientific rationality and formal logic', and the 'voice of the 'lifeworld', constructed through the intuitive, experiential perspective of the patient.

The presence of multiple 'voices' is, of course, not limited to medical consultations, but, as my brief analysis of the Tylenol package above illustrates, is a feature of nearly all communication around health and risk. The key questions for applied linguists when confronted with the multitude of 'voices' in texts and talk around health and risk are: How do we know when we are 'hearing' them? What concrete discursive features can we discern to distinguish one voice from another? How do these voices interact with one another, and what are the consequences of this interaction? And finally, who do these voices 'belong to' and whose interests do they serve? These are not just theoretical questions. They get to the heart not just of how doctors and patients negotiate medical consultations, but also of how people make sense of the multiple, often contradictory voices that speak to them about health and risk in their everyday lives.

The important thing about voices is that they constitute not just ways of talking, but ways of getting things done. Voices represent agendas, so that the doctor's way of speaking and of controlling what the patient is able to say both reflects what he or she is trying to do and actually contributes to *accomplishing* that agenda. Furthermore, it is through appropriating the 'voice of medicine' to accomplish these 'doctorly actions' that the doctor enacts his or her identity as a doctor and imputes to the patient the identity of a patient. Voices 'create "social positions" (perspectives) from which people are "invited" ("summoned") to speak, listen, act, read and write, think, feel, believe and value in certain characteristic, historically recognizable ways' (Gee, 1996, p. 128).

In the same way, the voices on the Tylenol package I discussed above are there to accomplish different kinds of actions – convincing me to buy the product, informing me about how to use it, warning me about its dangers, and indemnifying the company in the event that I suffer liver damage. Each of these actions creates for me a different social position in relation to the manufacturer. I am at once a customer, a patient, and a potential plaintiff.

Ultimately, then, interactions like medical consultations and texts like Tylenol packages involve complex dialogues not just between social actors (doctors and patients, manufacturers and customers) but also among the 'discourses' these actors give voice to and the institutions and groups which produce and reproduce these discourses. The speaker or writer is not just a social actor appropriating a voice, but 'the meeting point of many, sometimes conflicting, socially and historically defined Discourses' (Gee, 1996, p. 132). Therefore, when we ask 'who's speaking here?', we do not just mean 'is it the doctor or the patient?', or 'is it the corporation or the regulators that require certain information to be included on product packages?' although these socially constructed roles are usually associated with particular 'voices'. What we really mean is 'what *discourses* are being represented or "given voice to" by whom?'

Although Mishler did not intend through his analysis to imply that the physician speaks only with the 'voice of medicine' or that the 'voice of the lifeworld' is the sole province of the patient, there has been a tendency in subsequent studies of medical interactions to embrace this false dualism and to celebrate the 'voice of the lifeworld' as 'authentic' and denigrate the 'voice of medicine' as 'hegemonic'. In such analyses, as Atkinson (2009, para. 2.4) points out, the more the 'lifeworld' is celebrated as a 'true' reflection of the patient's experiences, the 'more the world of medicine is emptied of human, personal content', to the extent that such studies end up *constructing* these voices rather than actually 'hearing' them. Actual interactions are rarely so simple. Not only are the worlds of everyday life and medicine themselves made up of many competing voices, but participants in medical consultations as in other interactions also normally have a wide array of voices available to them, and sometimes the voice a particular speaker uses may not be entirely consistent with our expectations about their social role.

This fact was particularly apparent in a study I did in the late 1990s on the quality of life of people with HIV in Hong Kong (Jones et al., 2000), in which it was revealed that patients and medical personnel had very different ideas about what constituted appropriate ways of talking during medical consultations: HIV specialist doctors and nurses felt their patients were not communicative enough, especially when it came to discussing emotional problems or personal issues like sexual relationships, whereas their HIV positive patients sometimes found the medical staff nosey and intrusive. In other words, doctors and nurses worried that the 'voice of the lifeworld' was not sufficiently represented in consultations with these patients, whereas the patients preferred to stick with the 'voice of medicine'.

Part of the reason that the medical personnel in this context were concerned was that they assumed that these particular patients, because of their diagnosis, *must* be experiencing psychological or emotional problems, and if they weren't talking about them, they must be 'holding something back'. They felt that if their patients were not 'completely open' with them, it was much more difficult to provide them with the care they needed. One doctor in the study said, 'my interpretation [of a good relationship with an HIV positive patient] is that he is willing to open himself to you. You really have communication and trust with him.' Far from restricting themselves to the 'disinterested' perspective of the 'voice of medicine', many of these doctors viewed talk about 'lifeworld' issues as central to building and maintaining relationships of trust and essential for providing adequate care (especially when it came to monitoring their patients' compliance with complex medication regimens). Another factor contributing to doctors' willingness to invite the 'voice of the lifeworld' into their consultation rooms in this context was that, at that time, the number of patients diagnosed with HIV infection in Hong Kong was still relatively small, and HIV specialist medical personnel generally had more time to devote to each of their patients.

The patients in this study, on the other hand, viewed talk in medical contexts as more instrumental. When they reported talking to healthcare workers, the emphasis was on the practical nature of the talk and what it was meant to accomplish, such as better medication or relief from symptoms or side effects. As one patient put it when asked why she did not communicate more with the doctor, 'I don't have much to talk about with the doctor … I just go to get the medicine. If I have no pain, I just answer what he asks.' 'People always want to show concern for me,' said another. 'They're very nice, but I don't really want to talk to them.' For many of these patients, talking about personal matters to people outside of their circle of intimates was not generally part of their strategy for coping with HIV. That is not to say that they did not want to talk about their problems or the social and psychological pressures associated with HIV infection. They did, but they preferred to do so with friends, family members, or with other people living with HIV who could 'really understand' what they were talking about.

What these findings remind us is not just that different people may appropriate different voices, but that this appropriation is often highly strategic. The doctors in this study, for example, in promoting the 'voice of the lifeworld' were not abandoning the discourse of medicine, but rather, in part, appropriating the 'voice of the lifeworld' in the service of that discourse. Getting patients to talk about their experiences and feelings, they reasoned, was often the best way to discern things like whether or not they were taking their medications properly, the extent to which their symptoms and the side effects of the medicines were interfering with their normal functioning, and even the extent to which they were managing things like 'safer sex'. Similarly, for the patients, limiting talk of lifeworld issues in medical consultations was a strategic way of preventing the medical gaze from intruding too much into the lifeworld.

A similarly unstable relationship between voices and speakers can be seen in commercial texts like packages of over-the-counter medications and direct-to-consumer drug advertisements. The assumption of many is that manufacturers necessarily take up the 'voice of marketing', whereas government regulators impose upon such texts the 'voice of medicine' and the 'voice of the law' in the form of things like warning labels. Closer analysis of such texts, however (see for example Koteyko and Nerlich, 2007; Moses, 2000), reveals that manufacturers often appropriate the voice of medicine (in the form of charts and graphs and data from clinical studies), and the warnings of government regulators sometimes appropriate the rhetorical techniques of advertising to get customers' attention.

Among the most important contributions applied linguistics can offer the study of health and risk communication is to provide the analyst with a systematic way of actually 'hearing' these voices and identifying the various 'discourses' that they 'give voice' to. A number of scholars promoting applied linguistic approaches to health communication, including Cicourel (1992), Candlin and Candlin (2003), and Sarangi and Roberts (1999), have in fact argued that the task of understanding how larger social and institutional formations of power/knowledge are both reflected in and constituted through situated talk is one of the key challenges in the study of the discourse of health and risk. Studies which examine only the 'small d discourse' (Gee, 2011) of texts and interactions run the risk of focusing on what Lynch and Bogen (1994) have termed the 'disembodied utterance', and studies which seek to make grand pronouncements about 'capital D Discourses' without seeking out their instantiation in actual texts and talk risk not only 'making up' voices rather than 'hearing' them but also overemphasizing the hegemonic nature of discourses and ignoring the role of individual agency in people's actions around health and risk.

Applied linguistics offers a middle ground, giving us a way to explore how specific features of texts and interactions 'give voice' to broader macrostructures in the social formation (Fairclough, 1992a; Giddens, 1979; Marvel et al., 1999) and how these macrostructures enable and constrain the locally managed choices people make when they construct specific texts or engage in specific interactions (Candlin and Candlin, 2002; Hak, 1999).

As reflections of larger 'systems' of meaning, acting and being, voices carry with them rules or conventions governing their use and their relationship to other voices. These rules and conventions affect not just the lexico-grammatical, textual, and intertextual features of voices – the way they make certain formal features in texts and talk possible and preclude others – but also the circumstances into which they can be appropriated and the kinds of speakers and writers to whom they are available.

Voice appropriation and discourse representation

Fairclough (1992a) discusses two ways in which people represent the voices of others in texts and talk: what he calls *manifest intertextuality*, the appropriation of the actual words of specific people, and *constitutive intertextuality* (or *interdiscursivity*), the more subtle borrowing of different forms or styles of discourse (what Bakhtin calls *speech genres* and *social languages*). Manifest intertextuality is the much more straightforward and easily detected of the two. According to Fairclough (1992a), there are broadly two ways we can appropriate the actual words of others: either by placing boundaries around them, signaling through textual features like quotation marks and verbs of reporting that this voice is not our own, or by taking them up in ways that blur to various degrees the boundaries between the borrowed voice and our own voice, like paraphrase, presupposition, negation, metadiscourse, and irony. The ways speakers and writers manipulate the boundaries between their own words and the words of others conveys their attitude towards the voices they appropriate, and their relationship with other voices that are borrowed in the same text. They also, as Scollon (1998) points out, allow people to finely calibrate the claims and imputations of identity embodied in these acts of appropriation and adjust the level of participation they project for themselves in particular communities and institutions.

A good example of how people strategically align or distance themselves from others and claim for themselves certain social identities through manifest inter-textuality can be seen in Hamilton's (1998) study of the use of reported speech by members of an online community for survivors of bone marrow transplants and their relatives. In narratives about conflicts with medical personnel, Hamilton points out, people posting to the forum usually represent their own utterances or those of their relatives using indirect speech (paraphrase), whereas the voices of doctors are usually reported with direct speech (quotations). In a story told by the sister of a patient, for example, the sister writes:

> Susie mentioned that her mouth was getting really bad. Her doctor said, 'You think you feel bad now you haven't seen ANYTHING yet.'
>
> *(Hamilton, 1998, p. 63)*

Hamilton argues that one of the reasons contributors to the forum are more likely to directly quote the words of unhelpful physicians is to distance themselves from such voices and demonstrate (rather than just 'report') to readers the callousness of the physicians. This, however, is more than just a dramatic device. It is also a device, Hamilton suggests, for contributors to claim for themselves or their relatives social identities as 'survivors', people who are able not just to 'overcome … the disease' but also to 'surmount adversity in the form of unhelpful and unfeeling doctors' (p. 63).

Constitutive intertextuality or interdiscursivity is more difficult to detect. It refers to the borrowing not of the particular words of others, but of the styles, conventions, attitudes and perspectives of different 'discourses'. Fairclough mentions a number of features through which interdiscursivity can be detected in texts and talk, including the appropriation of genres (Bhatia, 1993; Swales, 1990), activity types (Levinson, 1979), rhetorical modes, and styles. Bakhtin (1986) divides these different kinds of 'voices' into two basic types: *speech genres* and *social languages*. Speech genres are the particular forms communication takes in various 'typical' circumstances. Solly (2007) gives an excellent example of the strategic mixing of genres in his analysis of a special advertising supplement for the *Guardian Weekly* called 'International Health' in which advertisements for expensive health insurance plans are embedded 'Trojan-horse style' (p. 30) in 'news articles'. Bakhtin (1981, p. 262) defines social languages as, 'social dialects, characteristic group behavior, professional jargons, generic languages, languages of generations and age groups, tendentious languages, languages of the authorities of various circles and of passing fashions, languages that serve the specific sociopolitical voices of the day'. As mentioned above, advertisements for health products like drugs and supplements often borrow features from the social language of doctors and researchers such as formulaic expressions like 'research shows', 'experts suggest', and 'studies have found' (Koteyko and Nerlich, 2007).

The different analytical perspectives in applied linguistics I discussed above offer different kinds of tools for the analysis of interdiscursivity, some focusing more on lexico-grammatical features, and others focusing more on ways voices are instantiated in broader forms of discourse. In analyzing texts, for example, we might focus on the ways voices are instantiated in specific linguistic features like the use of nominalization or the passive voice in scientific writing, or we might focus on the broader mixing of genres, as when conventions from pornography are appropriated into AIDS prevention discourse (Gilman, 1995; Patton, 1991). In interactions, 'voicing' might be accomplished through the appropriation of broad 'discourse types' which signal different activities, as in genetic counseling where, according to Sarangi (2000), informing, explaining, and advising are strategically mixed, or it might be accomplished through the moment-by-moment management of topics, turn taking, silences, and intonation.

Voices and power

Just being able to 'hear' voices, however, is not enough. It is also necessary to understand something about the relationship voices have to one another and the consequences their appropriation has on the concrete actions people are able to take. In this regard, Mishler was right when he noted that the overarching issue associated with voice appropriation in medical consultations is dominance. Others as well (P. Atkinson, 1995; Fairclough, 1992a; Todd and Fisher, 1993; Treichler, 1988a, 1988b) have also observed how voice appropriation functions as a means by which certain participants in interaction maintain their power over others, and, by extension, how certain groups, classes or professions maintain hegemonic control over certain domains of life.

Not only is the appropriation of particular 'voices' often restricted to particular people in interactions, but the way these voices function to define and constrain what counts as legitimate 'knowledge' can have the effect of marginalizing or rendering invisible certain social practices and social identities. This is particularly true in institutional interactions, such as the school placement meetings described by Mehan (1993), in which the 'voice of psychology' – ironically the one that was generated as a result of the least amount of actual contact with the child – ends up being regarded as more definitive than the observations of the child's teacher and even the experiences of the child's mother.

At the same time, it is also important to remember that voices can be appropriated in all sorts of strategic ways which might undermine rather than promote the ideologies of the discourses from which they come. While every word we speak is always 'half someone else's' (Bakhtin, 1981, p. 293), these words are also half 'our own', and when we borrow them, we 'populate' them with our own 'semantic and expressive intentions'. It is this interplay between the intentions of others embedded in the voices we borrow and our own intentions with which we populate these voices that, in the final analysis, ends up determining the kinds of social actions and social identities that these voices make possible.

Discourse and action

This brings me to the second problem that I believe applied linguistics can help to address in the study of health and risk communication: how to understand the relationship between discourse and social action. As I mentioned above, one of the things that separates applied linguistics from many other approaches to language and communication is its commitment to seeing language as a means for taking *action* rather than simply a means of transferring information from one person to another. As Bauman and Briggs (1990, p. 62) point out, however, 'to say that language use is social action is ... much easier than to develop frameworks that can identify and explain the nature of this dynamism.'

This problem of the relationship between discourse and action is, of course, central to the fields of clinical medicine and health promotion. For clinicians, so much of what they do is dependent on transforming action into discourse and discourse back into action. Signs, symptoms, biological processes and patients' past actions are transformed through examinations and medical tests into *texts*: lab results, medical histories, images of bodily organs, and, eventually diagnoses, which themselves are then transformed back into action: treatments. In each step along the way, the ability of certain actions (such as conducting a test) to yield appropriate forms of discourse (a result from which a plausible diagnosis can be arrived at), and the ability of discourse (such as an explanation of a recommended course of treatment) to yield the right kind of action (patient adherence to a regimen of medication), are critical factors in whether or not a patient improves. Similarly, the central task of health promoters is to make sense of the actions of particular people around particular health issues and to determine what kinds of discursive interventions are most likely to result in behavior change.

Understanding the relationship between discourse and action is also central to the everyday lives of laypeople as they attempt to manage their own actions (related to things like smoking, diet, and exercise), and to make sense of the myriad, sometimes contradictory discourses they encounter telling them what they should and should not do. The traditional way health educators and medical practitioners have viewed the relationship between discourse and action is based on the underlying assumption that discourse leads (or should lead) rather directly and unproblematically to some kind of desired action. The 'better' the discourse (in the form of information) the better the health outcomes. Unfortunately, things do not always work out that way. In fact, time and time again in the area of health and risk we are confronted with situations in which the relationship between what is said, written, or otherwise communicated and what people actually do is complicated, indirect, or utterly contrary to what is expected.

One way to understand the relationship between discourse and action is to adopt the position of Scollon and his colleagues (Norris and Jones, 2005; Scollon, 2001b), itself adapted from Vygotsky (1962), and consider discourse as a *mediational means* through which action is carried out. For Vygotsky, all actions (including individual mental functioning) are mediated through *cultural tools*, which have the effect of amplifying and constraining what we are able to do. He divided these tools into physical or 'technological' tools (syringes, stethoscopes, condoms and other material objects) and psychological or 'semiotic' tools, a category which includes 'language; various systems for counting; mnemonic techniques; algebraic symbol systems; works of art; writing; schemes, diagrams, maps, and mechanical drawings; [and] all sorts of conventional signs'. In terms of discourse, we need to account for both its material *and* its semiotic qualities. What we are able to do with discourse is, on one hand, determined by the materiality of texts, the way they exist in time and space (the actions that can be taken with an electronic medical record, for example, are very different from those that can be taken with a paper one (Iedema, 2003b)), and, on the other hand, determined by the semiotic aspects of discourse, that is, how we are able represent the world, how we are able to construct relationships with those with whom we are communicating, and how we are able to organize our meanings in ways that make sense to other people (Halliday, 1973). Such aspects of discourse include not just the lexicogrammatical resources of whatever semiotic system we happen to be using, but also how these resources go into making up the 'voices' (speech genres and social languages) that are available to us to perform certain activities and enact certain identities. Focusing on mediation gives us a way to avoid naïvely considering the discourse alone and wondering why it does not lead to the actions it was intended to lead to, or naïvely considering the social actors alone and wondering why 'those people are acting so irrationally', and to instead focus on the 'tension' (Wertsch, 1994) between what discourse allows people to do and what they actually do with it as they appropriate and adapt it in the service of specific social goals.

The idea of *mediation* helps us stake out a kind of middle ground in the contentious debate in social theory over the respective roles of structure and agency in the lives of individuals (Turner, 1992), in which macro-theorists have traditionally emphasized structure and those who take a micro-perspective have emphasized individual agency (Lupton, 2003). From the perspective of mediation, agency is always *negotiated*, in the actual performance of *mediated actions*, between social actors (with their individual goals and plans) and social structures (which enable and constrain certain actions through the cultural tools they make available).

It is not enough, however, to understand how discourse affects action; it is also necessary to understand how action *creates* discourse. Actions and discourse exist in complex historical chains that stretch out over time and across contexts; it is often the discourse that is produced through one set of actions that makes subsequent actions possible. This complex chaining of texts and actions is illustrated by Mehan (1993) in his description of how the diagnosis of a 'learning disability' is accomplished over time as the actions from one setting in a sequence of events (a classroom encounter) are transformed into a text (a form filled out by the teacher), which is later used in a subsequent event (a school appraisal meeting), which generates a new text (a 'summary of recommendations'), which can then be used to take subsequent actions (the placement of a student in a special class). Through this process of actions being transformed into texts and texts being used to take actions, Mehan argues, the child becomes increasingly objectified. As Scollon (2001b) would put it, through these cycles of discourse and action, the child is increasingly 'technologized' as a certain kind of child (a recognizable 'social identity') and the actions of managing the child become 'technologized' as a certain kind of 'social practice'. What Scollon (see also Jones, 2002a; Scollon, 2001b) means by 'technologization' is the process whereby, through these repeated cycles of discourse and action, social identities and social practices become solidified, conventionalized, and take on the status of 'technologies' that can be lifted out of one context and transported into another. As these technologies are taken up in subsequent actions, the social actions and social identities associated with them often become harder and harder to resist.

Iedema (2001a) makes this point in his study of the chain of discourse and action associated with the renovation of a mental hospital in New South Wales in which representations of practices and identities migrate over the course of the project from spoken discourse in meetings, to written plans, to blueprints, and finally to the actual brick and mortar of the hospital wing. As meanings move through increasingly durable forms of discourse, Iedema argues, they become more and more difficult to negotiate and change: the 'hold' that discourse has on the actual actions people are able to take becomes increasingly strong. Scollon (2001a) makes a similar point in his analysis of what he calls the 'funnel of commitment' (see chapter 5), which he illustrates by considering the chain of discourse and action involved in having a cup of coffee in Starbucks. As the chain of events leading up to actually drinking the cup of coffee progresses from entering the shop, to choosing an item and placing the order, to paying, to picking up the finished cup of coffee, this chain becomes increasingly difficult to reverse.

Although architectural planning and having a cup of coffee may at first seem to have little to do with health and risk communication, these two studies illustrate a number of important points in understanding how discourse affects the actions we take around health. First, they show how actions are 'threaded together' in various ways by the discourse that we produce. Second, they show how the form this discourse takes plays a big role in determining the kinds of actions that we can take and our ability to reverse a chain of actions once it is initiated. Finally, these two studies show how sometimes discourse not directly related to an individual's health like meeting minutes, architectural plans, and menus in coffee shops may, some-where down the chain of actions, actually have a profound impact on health: when you think about it, what could be more important for health than whether or not a hospital gets built or whether or not we are able to resist that next cup of coffee, that next piece of cake, or that next cigarette?

Entextualization and recontextualization

The challenge for applied linguists is to understand the *discursive processes* through which social actions and social actors are transformed into social practices and social identities, and the processes involved in appropriating these practices and identities (and the texts necessary to perform them) into different social contexts.

Bauman and Briggs (1990) refer to these two kinds of processes as *entextualization* and *recontextualization*. Entextualization involves the various mechanisms through which actions are turned into discourse. The most important thing about entex-tualization is its role in the 'technologization' of social practices and social identities, the way it makes practices and identities more and more 'solid', and often more and more difficult to resist or question. It is the process through which, as Mehan (1993, p. 243) puts it, 'the clarity of social facts such as "intelligence", "deviance", "health", and "illness" [is] produced from the ambiguity of everyday life.' Recon-textualization refers to the often strategic ways these technologized practices and identities are appropriated into specific 'sites of engagement' (Jones, 2005c; Scollon, 2001b) to take specific actions such as deciding on a course of medical treatment, taking time off to be with a sick relative, regulating what one's children eat, or negotiating sexual contact.

Both our individual social lives and the lives of the institutions, communities, and cultures in which we live take place through cycles of entextualization and recontextualization in which our actions produce discourse and discourse is

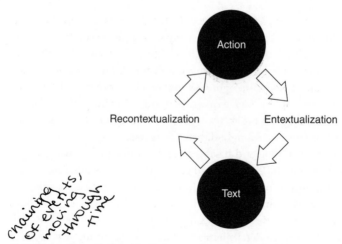

chaining of events/ moving through time

FIGURE 2.1 The relationship between discourse and action

appropriated to take new actions (see Figure 2.1). Analyzing a single text or a single moment of social interaction in the absence of an understanding of where this discourse came from and what might happen to it in the future can often tell us very little about what people are actually able to do with it at that moment. Scollon (2008) calls the historical pathways formed by these chains of discourse and action 'discourse itineraries', and he argues that the primary task of discourse analysts is not to extract discourse from these itineraries, but rather to follow it through the complex displacements that work 'across a wide variety of times, places, people, media, and objects' (p. 233).

While questions about 'entextualization', 'recontextualization', and the 'techno-logization of practice' may at first seem rather theoretical, as I pointed out above, these processes have direct practical relevance for health and risk. My 'reading' of the Tylenol box with which I began this chapter depends crucially on the inter-section of multiple discourse itineraries, itineraries involving my personal history of pain and pain reliever use, itineraries involving corporate decision-making and marketing strategies, itineraries involving scientific research and court cases, and even itineraries involving the stocking of particular products in airport shops. All of these historical trajectories came together to make the action of me buying that box of Tylenol in San Francisco possible.

Action and power

Like the issue of voice appropriation which I considered above, entextualization and recontextualization are ultimately a matter of power. According to Bauman and Briggs (1990, p. 76), 'To decontextualize and recontextualize a text is ... an act of control, and in regard to the differential exercise of such control the issue of social power arises.' Such power is a function of who has access to different texts and different resources for entextualization, the different claims to legitimacy they have to entextualize and recontextualize texts, different competencies involved in the process of entextualization and the appropriation of texts, and different values attached to different types of texts in various communities and institutions. Anyone who has tried to navigate their way through the cycles of entextualization and recontextualization involved in things like seeking emergency medical care, managing a chronic condition, making an insurance claim, or participating in a program of recovery like Alcoholics Anonymous knows how important questions about who is allowed to author what kinds of texts and what they are allowed to do with them can be.

*

In the following chapters I will proceed to develop the analytical tools that I introduced above, beginning in the next chapter with a consideration of different processes of *entextualization* and how they contribute to the 'technologization' of social practices and social identities around health and risk.

3

ENTEXTUALIZING HEALTH AND RISK

In February of 1998 the British medical journal *The Lancet* published an article by Dr Andrew Wakefield and his colleagues (Wakefield et al., 1998) claiming to have identified a possible link between autism and the combined measles, mumps, rubella (MMR) vaccine. Although the paper was published under the heading 'early report' and accompanied by an article critiquing its assertions (Chen and DeStefano, 1998), soon after its publication the 'debate' about the safety of the MMR vaccine escalated into a full-blown media controversy in Britain, a controversy that quickly spread to other countries. More than a decade later doubts about the safety of MMR and other childhood vaccinations continues to affect vaccination rates in Europe, the United States and Australasia, despite that fact that no credible link has ever been found between vaccinations and autism (Donald and Muthu, 2002; Smith et al., 2008).

One thing that has kept this controversy alive over the years is the proliferation of personal stories from parents whose children developed symptoms of autism shortly after having the vaccinations, stories that have been printed in newspapers, broadcast on television, and reported on numerous websites that invite readers to respond to them with their own narratives. The effectiveness of these stories in convincing people of the link between MMR and autism lies in part in how similar they are, the way they reproduce the pattern of countless other stories by countless other parents about their children's 'transformation'. As anti-vaccine activist Shelley Reynolds noted in her testimony to the US government committee investigating vaccination policy, 'It's always the same story: Child is normal, child gets a vaccine, child disappears within days or weeks into the abyss of autism' (Mnookin, 2011, p. 142).

In the debate about the safety of vaccines, the relentless accumulation of these 'real life' stories of parents has often overshadowed the rational arguments of doctors and public health officials. In fact, by responding to these stories with 'facts' and statistics, the biomedical community often ends up portraying itself as undermining the 'real world' experience of parents with 'dry generalizations and abstract data' (Speers and Lewis, 2004, p. 177) – Mishler's clash between the 'voice of medicine' and the 'voice of the lifeworld' played out on the media stage. One reason, in fact, that the portrayal of the government and medical authorities 'not listening' to the experiences of parents has been so rhetorically effective for vaccine opponents is its resonance with many people's own experiences of 'not being listened to' by their doctors. Wakefield himself frequently appropriated this storyline in portraying himself as different from other doctors. In response to criticisms of his Lancet article, for example, he said: 'the approach of the clinical scientists should reflect the first and most important lesson learnt as a medical student – to listen to the patient or the patient's parent, and they will tell you the answer' (Wakefield, 1998, p. 908).

*

The conflict between scientists and anti-vaccine activists described above is not just one between two different opinions regarding a medical issue, nor is it simply an argument between 'experts' (who 'know what they are talking about') and 'laypeople' (who 'don't'). It is more fundamentally a conflict between two different ways of entextualizing reality, each with different ways of organizing information and different ways of creating relationships between the producers and consumers of texts. The parents of autistic children and the journalists who recorded their experiences spoke in *stories*, complete with characters, conflict, and pathos. The scientists, on the other hand, spoke in arguments, marshaling evidence from a large number of anonymous cases to assess the validity of a particular proposition. It would be a mistake to dismiss either of these ways of entextualizing reality as less legitimate than the other: both have a long history in the health sciences and both are, in their own ways, empirically grounded: the stories of the parents are as 'real' as the clinical trials of the scientists, and vice versa.

In this chapter I will examine how the *entextualization* of health-related knowledge and experiences in artifacts such as medical case reports, health promotion pamphlets, pharmaceutical advertisements, scientific papers, and popular presentations of medical information in the media can affect the way people think and act about health and risk. One important aspect of this is the way knowledge changes as it moves from one genre to another, being subjected to the conventions of entextualization of different 'discourse communities' (Swales, 1990). Considerable attention has been paid to the 'popularization' of medical discourse as it moves from the more specialized genres of physicians and researchers to mainstream media, genres like newspaper articles, TV documentaries, and internet web pages. Equally important, however, is the way the experiences and understandings of 'ordinary' people are interpreted and transformed by 'experts'.

Scientists, healthcare workers, and health promoters often express dismay at the way media 'oversimplify' or 'distort' medical information, and incidents like the MMR controversy I described above are held up as examples (Ramsay et al., 2002; Speers and Lewis, 2004). Criticisms of media portrayals of scientific and medical knowledge, however, can sometimes traffic in their own brand of distortion. Cook and his colleagues (Cook, 2004; Cook et al., 2004), for example, in their study of public debates around genetically modified food, found that scientists often exaggerate the inaccuracy of media accounts about science, underestimate the ability of the public to understand scientific information, and themselves resort to dramatic anecdotes and sensationalist metaphors (such as comparing anti-GM activists to 'terrorists'). In other words, while scientists accuse the media of oversimplifying science, they themselves often oversimplify the professional practices of journalists and the everyday 'sense-making' practices of non-scientists.

Just as the popular accounts of the MMR vaccine controversy described above sometimes portray it as a clash between the 'real life' experiences of parents and the 'cold', abstract arguments of scientists, scientific accounts of the media popularization of science often portray it as a clash between the 'real knowledge' of science and the 'perverted' knowledge of ordinary people (Weingart, 1998). Suhardja (2009) calls this way of talking about media popularizations of scientific knowledge 'the discourse of distortion'. According to this discourse, any difference between 'genuine' science and popularized science is necessarily the result of 'distortion' or 'degradation' of the facts (Hilgartner, 1990, p. 519).

One problem with the 'discourse of distortion' is that it equates 'popularization' with 'simplification'. Analyses of the process of popularization of technical discourse from an applied linguistic perspective (see, for example, Beacco et al., 2002; Calsamiglia and van Dijk, 2004; Moirand, 2003), however, have revealed a very different picture. Not only does popularization involve complex linguistic and rhetorical strategies such as metaphorization, exemplification, and reformulation, designed to help readers to make links between what they already know and the new information that is being presented, but the texts that result are often extremely sophisticated attempts to explore not just the scientific aspects of an issue but also its social, political, economic, and ethical aspects.

Rather than speaking of 'simplification' or 'distortion', a more useful way to understand what is involved when different kinds of people construct texts about health and risk is through understanding not just the different 'knowledge' and experiences these people have, but also the different resources they have for *entextualizing* their knowledge and experiences, and the role these processes of entextualization have in constructing and maintaining social practices and social identities around health and risk.

Texts and the discursive construction of health and risk

When most applied linguists refer to 'texts' they mean any kind of coherent discourse, written, spoken, graphic, or multimodal. Texts include, in Iedema's (2001a, p. 187) words, not just 'books, films and television shows', but also 'birthday parties, interviews, telephone calls and football games'. In this chapter and the next, however, I will be making a distinction between texts as bounded, 'portable' pieces of discourse that can be transported from one place and time to another and 'interactions', which take place at particular times and in particular places, which I will be referring to in the next chapter as 'sites of engagement' (Scollon, 2001a). In a sense, Iedema makes a similar distinction when he refers to 'birthday parties and telephone calls and the like' which 'take place in real time and space' as 'presentations', and books, films and television shows which construct times and spaces using the logic of the media through which they are expressed as 're-presentations'. Texts, as Phillips and his colleagues (2004, p. 638) put it, allow thoughts and actions to transcend 'the essentially transitory character of social processes' and to cross 'separate and diverse local settings'. In so doing, they play a particularly important role in producing and maintaining the social categories and practices that shape our understandings of health and risk across diverse social settings.

Texts and interactions, as I noted in the last chapter, are related to each other along what Scollon (2008) refers to as 'itineraries of discourse'. People regularly appropriate texts into their interactions and interactions typically generate more texts. It is through these cycles of entextualization and recontextualization that people 'technologize' social practices and social identities, 'talking' their social worlds into existence.

Texts and entextualization

In the last chapter I borrowed the terminology of linguistic anthropologists Bauman and Briggs (1990), calling the process through which texts are created *entextualization*, and the process through which they are appropriated into new situations *recontextualization*. Bauman and Briggs (1990) define entextualization as 'the process of rendering discourse extractable, of making a stretch of linguistic production into a unit – a text – that can be lifted out of its interactional setting' (p. 73).

Entextualization is the fundamental process through which we 'make sense' of the world. It is the way isolated actions bounded by time and space come to be regarded as social practices, the way individuals come to be recognized as certain types of people, and the way groups of individuals come to be seen as communities, institutions or nations. It is through texts that 'diseases', 'disabilities', 'doctors', and 'patients' come into being. Ian Hacking (1986) captures this central epistemological truth when he writes, 'if new modes of description come into being, new possibilities for action come into being in consequence' (p. 231).

Along with describing social actors and social practices symbolically, texts also instantiate them materially, and this materiality of texts contributes to the 'solidification' of social practices and social identities. As Iedema (2001b, p. 24) points out, entextualization invariably involves 'resemiotization' (see p. 36) in which 'more temporal meaning-making, such as talk and gesture' is translated into more 'durable' and *propagative* kinds of meaning-making, such as printed reports, designs, and ... buildings' (see also Latour and Woolgar, 1986). This process, Iedema argues, has the effect of distancing the social actors and social actions represented in texts from the social interactions that actually created them, of 'stabilizing meaning' and of 'reinventing' concrete, situated actions as 'specialized and authoritative discourses' (p. 32).

Finally, the power of texts to 'technologize' or, in Hacking's parlance, to 'make up' people and practices has to do not just with their ability to represent social actions and social actors and to materialize social practices, but also with their ability to hold together complex chains of social actions and to sustain social practices and social identities across time and space. Texts create constancy across times, spaces, and groups of people (Barton and Hamilton, 2005, p. 23). They link together disparate events, actions, people, and organizations through the 'discourse itineraries' along which they travel.

In what follows I will discuss five processes of entextualization, how these processes function as *resources* with which people communicate about health and risk, and how they contribute to the *technologization* of social identities and social practices. These processes are:

(1) *lexicalization* (including naming and classification, metaphorization and quantification) – the process through which *things* (objects, people, concepts) are labeled and the world is divided up and epistemologically structured;

(2) *grammaticalization* – the process through which objects, people and concepts are portrayed as interacting with one another to perform various *actions* and enact various states of affairs;

(3) *personalization* – the process through which *relationships* between 'readers' and 'writers' are constructed and notions of certainty, doubt, choice and obligation are negotiated;

(4) *organization* – the process through which texts are *structured* around the cognitive schemata of individuals and the communicative goals of communities and institutions;

(5) *resemiotization* – the process through which meanings are translated from one semiotic system to another.

Lexicalization

Perhaps the most obvious way people represent reality is in the words they choose to 'stand for' different things, people, ideas, events and actions. Words and the ways they are related through, for example, synonymy, hyponymy and antonymy (Fairclough, 1989) construct systems of inclusion and exclusion (Gee, 1996) that divide up the world in particular ways. I will be referring to this process of labeling and division as *lexicalization*.

Lexicalization is not just a matter of labeling something, but also of situating that thing within a 'larger linguistic structuring' (Berger and Luckmann, 1967) in which it exists in specific relationships with other things. These systems of categorization are socially formed and culturally transmitted resources that people draw upon to make sense of the world and to engage in various forms of everyday and professional reasoning. They become so interwoven with everyday and institutional practices that, apart from meeting classificatory needs, they 'become part of how individuals conduct themselves and enact their social identities' (Sarangi, 2000; Sarangi and Candlin, 2003, p. 118; see also Mehan, 1993). Doctors, for example, draw upon systems of categorization of diseases in order to decide on a diagnosis and course of treatment, as well as to enact their professional identities, and laypeople draw upon their own systems of categorization in deciding what kinds of activities, foods, mind-altering substances, or sexual partners are 'safe' and what kinds are 'dangerous', and in so doing also show themselves to be certain kinds of people.

The power of classification is perhaps nowhere more evident than in the profession of medicine, which is predicated upon practices of naming and categorizing diseases. In his essay 'The Importance of a Theory of Signs and a Critique of Language in the Study of Medicine' (1923), epidemiologist Dr F. G. Crookshank notes that 'under the influence of certain schools of thought, and certain habits of expression, we have become accustomed to speak and write as if a disease were a natural object', and that 'no great advance is probable in the domain of Medicine until the belief in the real existence of diseases is abandoned.'

What Dr Crookshank is getting at is the fact that all diseases are socially constructed. Whether or not this process of construction impedes medical advances or is what makes them possible, of course, is a matter of some debate. Many would argue that it is the process of naming and classifying diseases and conditions, and of assigning to them certain symptoms and etiology, that makes them 'manageable', and, ultimately, treatable. At the heart of this debate is the fact that the act of naming (or not naming) a phenomenon always brings along with it certain affordances and constraints on how we can think of and act in relation to it, not only highlighting certain aspects of the phenomenon and obscuring others, but fixing that phenomenon into a larger epistemological system which is inevitably associated with a particular ideology or the interests of a particular group. In medicine these epistemological systems are made explicit in documents like the *International Statistical Classification of Diseases and Related Health Problems* (ICD) published by the World Health Organization and the *Diagnostic and Statistical Manual of Mental Disorders* (*DSM*) published by the American Psychiatric Association. Texts such as these lay out the symptoms and signs that physicians use to assign a particular disease to a particular patient. They are linked to other texts such as interview schedules, examination protocols, and laboratory assays to help construct the *social practice* of diagnosis (see chapter 6).

All such systems of classification are, by their very nature, *ad hoc*, subject to change as scientific knowledge advances and the politics of scientific research and public health policy plays out. Biomedical history is full of famous examples of the evolution of disease names and diagnostic criteria. The preferred name for tuberculosis, for example, changed three times over the course of a few decades in the nineteenth century from 'phthisis' to 'consumption' to 'tuberculosis'. Such revisions are often the result of the inventions of new 'technologies of entextualization' (Jones, 2009a,

p. 29), which make possible new ways of experiencing and describing the world. It was, for example, Laennec's invention of the stethoscope that made the diagnosis of 'phthisis' possible, and Robert Koch's 1882 discovery of the staining technique to make *mycobacterium tuberculosis* visible under a microscope that made infection with the bacteria a criterion for the diagnosis of tuberculosis.

The way diseases are classified and labeled, however, is often as much a matter of changes in institutional and professional practices as of advances in scientific knowledge. Mayes and Horwitz (2005, p. 249), for example, argue that the transformation in the late 1970s in the way the *DSM* defined mental illnesses from 'broad, etiologically defined entities ... to symptom-based, categorical diseases' was the result not of increased scientific understanding of these diseases, but of pressure from insurance companies and the pharmaceutical industry to make the classification system more amiable to practices of reporting, billing, and marketing. More recent changes in the *DSM* played an important role in suspicions about the relationship between the MMR vaccine and autism. One of the major pieces of 'evidence' anti-vaccine activists use to support their claims that vaccinations cause autism is the rapid rise in autism diagnoses following the introduction of the vaccination in Britain in 1988. This increase, however, is more likely to have been caused by a change in the system for classifying autism itself (Wing and Potter, 2002). Whereas the previous *DSM*-III, released in 1980, listed only six symptoms, in the new *DSM*-IV, released in 1984, the list of possible symptoms was increased to sixteen (Mnookin, 2011).

Metaphorization

One of the most widely studied forms of lexicalization in health and risk communication is metaphorization. Like other forms of labeling, metaphors work to construct reality by fixing an object, person or phenomenon into 'a coherent network of entailments that highlight some features of reality and hide others' (Lakoff and Johnson, 1980, p. 157). What is unique about metaphors is that they unite disparate domains of experience, causing the knowledge, feelings, and sets of expectations associated with one domain to be transferred to the other.

Perhaps the most famous treatment of metaphor in the discourse of health is the work of Susan Sontag, most notably her 1977 *Illness as Metaphor* and her later *AIDS and Its Metaphors* (1988) (published together in 1991). Sontag claims that in every age particular diseases become charged with meaning by being metaphorically associated with other spheres of human existence like war, morality, and sexuality, and that eventually these diseases themselves become metaphors for what societies at particular times most fear. By far the most common metaphor for illness, Sontag points out, is 'disease is war', manifested as descriptions of diseases 'invading the society', and efforts to cure them referred to as 'fights', and 'battles'. Such metaphors, she argues, can have a profoundly demoralizing effect on people who are suffering from diseases like cancer and AIDS. Reisfield and Wilson (2004, p. 4024) give a particularly vivid example of this in their account of the aggressive language used by a doctor to describe a planned cancer treatment to a patient (who later chose to change physicians):

> I'm going to kill you. Everyday, I'm going to kill you, and then I'm going to bring you back to life. We're going to hit you with chemo, and then hit you again, and hit you again. You're not going to be able to walk. We're practically going to have to teach you to walk again after we're done.

Sontag's work focuses primarily on the distorting nature of metaphors, arguing that they inject ideology and morality into discussions that should be 'objective' and 'scientific'. One problem with this position is that scientific discourse itself depends heavily on metaphor. Van-Rijn-van Tongeren (1997) in her corpus-based study of metaphors in medical texts, for example, reveals that many of the metaphors for cancer which Sontag considers 'unscientific' (such as cancer is war, cancer cells are animals, and cancer is the enigma in a detective story) are actually used quite frequently by scientists, and that in the context of scientific genres they sometimes function as aids in the formulation of theories and hypotheses (see also Boyd, 1993; Knudsen, 2003).

Another problem is that even in the context of popular discourse about health and disease, metaphors do not always have the stigmatizing or disempowering effects Sontag associates with them. For some patients the military metaphor for cancer, for instance, can actually be enabling, inspiring resolve (Reisfield and Wilson, 2004). Metaphors can also have useful explanatory powers: popular portrayals of medical knowledge often use simple metaphors from everyday domains like plumbing and electronics to explain medical procedures or the workings of the human body (Banks and Thompson, 1996). Such uses of metaphor, rather than acts of 'distortion', should actually be seen as sophisticated rhetorical practices designed to facilitate explanation, elaboration, or clarification. In their study of popular presentations of genomics, Calsamiglia and van Dijk (2004) highlight the challenges of formulating suitable metaphors for explaining scientific concepts to laypeople, arguing that writers must take into account readers' previous experiences in a wide range of domains as well as understand the fundamental cognitive categories they use to organize knowledge. Some, in fact, have argued that the problem of communicating medical knowledge to laypeople is not one of too much metaphor, but of too little. Hanne and Hawken (2007, p. 97), for example, recommend that 'a richer fund of metaphors' be developed for educating people about cardiovascular disease and facilitating physician–patient communication about it.

Quantification

Another important form of lexicalization in health and risk communication is *quantification*. Quantification is, as Potter and his colleagues put it, a process by which objects and concepts are '*constituted* through linking them to numbers' (Potter et al., 1991, p. 337). What is being achieved through quantification, they argue, is not just the operation of 'counting' certain things, but also the act of deciding which things 'count'.

While in the minds of most laypeople the association of health sciences with quantification has become naturalized, the preoccupation with quantification in medicine is actually a rather recent phenomenon. For most of the history of Western medicine, clinical practice has been a decidedly qualitative affair, and in the nineteenth and early twentieth centuries many physicians actively resisted the introduction of quantification into their work. In 1837, for example, eminent French physician Francois Double argued in a debate at the French Academy of Medicine that the introduction of mathematical models into diagnostic decision-making would reduce the physician to 'a shoemaker who after having measured the feet of a thousand persisted in fitting everyone based on an imaginary model' (Chen, 2003, p. 6). It was only after World War II that physicians began regularly dealing in measurement and statistics, and randomized clinical trials were not widely used for assessing medical interventions until the 1960s (Matthews, 1995).

With advances in medical technologies that can measure with great accuracy things like bone density and blood cholesterol levels and statistical methods that can predict the likelihood of disease occurrence in individuals and populations, more and more communication around health and risk makes use of quantification. This increased reliance on quantification has ushered in a new way of practicing medicine, commonly referred to as *evidence-based medicine* (B. Brown et al., 2006; Evidence-Based Medicine Working Group, 1992), in which physicians' decisions are based not on their own experiences or preferences but on the aggregated results of clinical trials. 'Good health', for both healthcare professionals and laypeople, has increasingly become less of an embodied experience and more of an abstract, calculative exercise, with physicians increasingly 'treating the numbers' – prescribing drugs or other treatments to patients based on laboratory tests rather than physical symptoms (McDonald, 1996) – and public health campaigns, especially around conditions like coronary heart disease, increasingly framing 'good health' as a matter of 'knowing your numbers' (see for example Ma et al., 2011).

Perhaps the chief difference between quantification and other forms of lexicalization is that, in a society dominated by what Scollon and his colleagues (Scollon et al., 2012) call 'the Utilitarian discourse system', it is afforded a special 'epistemological authority' (Danisch and Mudry, 2008, p. 130), an authority that derives from the belief that numbers are 'ideologically neutral' and immune to human bias. As a result, when confronted with hard-to-understand statistics people seldom question them and often blame their inability to understand them on their own ignorance. Like other processes of entextualization, however, quantification is not a neutral reflection of reality, but a *rhetorical device* that is used to make some aspects of reality criterial and obscure others. Discourse analysts like Potter and his colleagues (1991) have given numerous examples of how expressions of quantification are deployed strategically in the support of various social or institutional agendas. They observe, for example, how the selection of proportions or percentages (1 out of 100 or 1%), 'precise' figures or approximations (9.63% vs. 'close to ten percent'), and different orders of magnitude (250,000 vs. 'a quarter of a million'), can be used to make values seem smaller or larger, or to represent contrasts as either extreme or negligible. There are, however, even more fundamental issues surrounding the rhetorical nature of quantification, issues about the communication of *what* has been counted, *how* it has been counted, and *why* it has been counted.

The psychologist Gerd Gigerenzer (2002) argues that the confusion that many people associate with expressions of quantification, especially when it comes to probabilities, is essentially a matter of grammatical reference: the *reference set* which many of these expressions refer to is often ambiguous. One example he gives is a patient being informed that he has a 30% to 50% chance of experiencing sexual dysfunction after taking Prozac and wondering if this means that 30% to 50% of the people who take the drug experience sexual dysfunction or that he will experience sexual dysfunction in 30% to 50% of his own sexual encounters. Gigergenzer notes that patients who are given this information in 'natural frequencies' (3 to 5 people out of 10 who take this drug experience sexual problems), are more likely to opt for the treatment. Similarly, a parent who is told that her child is more than 2.5 times more likely to have a febrile seizure following the MMR vaccine might be duly alarmed, especially since it is unclear what the reference set is. She might assume that this means that children who have the vaccine are 2.5 times more likely to have febrile seizures than children who do not. What it actually means is that children who have the vaccine are 2.5 times more likely to experience febrile seizures *following* the vaccine than at other times. However, the overall increase of febrile seizures in vaccine recipients is less than 2 per 1,000 children (Vestergaard et al., 2004), fewer than would be expected among children who have actually contracted measles.

As I noted above, things like diseases and demographic groups do not exist as independent entities. They are discursively constructed based on agreed-upon criteria, which are subject to change as the result of such things as technological advances and the political and economic agendas of certain groups. The same is true for the criteria for quantifying various medical conditions. Statements about the rising rates of obesity in the United States or the characterization of a patient as having 'high cholesterol', for example, obscure the complex of often contentious negotiations within and across scientific bodies, government bureaus, and insurance and pharmaceutical companies that go into deciding what counts as obese and what level of cholesterol counts as high. In a now famous article on the quantitative definition of medical conditions, Schwartz and Woloshin (1999) describe how recommendations by professional bodies in the 1990s for revising quantitative thresholds for conditions such as diabetes, hypertension, high cholesterol, and obesity had the effect of increasing the number of cases of these conditions in the United States by nearly 155 million and ultimately labeling 75 percent of the US population as 'diseased'. Sales of drugs for these four conditions have represented the bulk of the profits of pharmaceutical companies since these revisions were adopted (Moynihan and Cassels, 2005).

Many expressions of quantification in health-related texts are also notoriously unclear about *how things have been counted*. When a woman over 50 is told that having an annual mammogram reduces her risk of dying from breast cancer by

25 percent, this is an expression of *relative risk* – a comparison of the number of women dying of breast cancer who did receive mammography (3 out of 1,000) with the number of those who did not (4 out of 1,000). The absolute risk reduction in this case is only 0.01 percent (Gigerenzer, 2002; Rifkin et al., 2006). Expressing risk in relative terms is a popular strategy in media texts, where it makes for more dramatic headlines; in advertisements from pharmaceutical companies, where it makes the products advertised appear more effective; and in grant application and research reports, where it makes the results of studies seem more significant.

Finally, expressions of quantification often mask the social and institutional processes behind decisions as to why some things are counted and others are not. In her book *The Wisdom of Whores* (2008) about HIV epidemiology, Elizabeth Pisani talks about the practice among workers in AIDS organizations in the late 1990s of 'beating up' statistics about the spread of HIV in the 'general population' in order to convince conservative governments in Asia and Latin America, which were less interested in devoting resources to a disease that affected mostly gay men, IV drug users, and prostitutes, to step up prevention efforts. One example of this practice she gives comes from the 1998 UNAIDS report she authored:

> [In India] the virus is firmly embedded in the general population among women whose only risk behavior is having sex with their own husbands. In a study of nearly 400 women attending STD clinics in Pune, 93% were married and 91% had never had sex with anyone but their husband, All of these women were infected with a sexually transmitted disease, and a shocking 13.6% of them tested positive for HIV.
>
> *(Pisani, 2008, p. 28)*

As Pisani points out, while the numbers reported are accurate, they present a much more dire picture than actually existed. First, the figures came from one small study focusing only on women who had already been diagnosed with sexually transmitted diseases, and, second, most of the women were probably married to men who visited prostitutes, which is actually a small minority of Indian men. 'They didn't represent the "general population" in any way,' she writes. 'But the way I wrote it pretty much implied that HIV was raging through the faithful wives of India' (Pisani, 2008, p. 28). As this example demonstrates, the ideological dimension of quantitative expressions lies not just in their tendency to obscure how things are counted, but also in their tendency to reproduce ideological notions of what is 'worth counting': this passage both exploits and reinforces the idea that married women 'count' more than prostitutes, and that they 'count' as members of the 'general population', whereas prostitutes, gay men, and IV drug users do not.

Grammaticalization

I use the term *grammaticalization* to refer to the way words are joined together to form what Gee (2011) calls 'who's-doing-whats', representations of particular actors *doing things* to, with, and for each other. Like lexicalization, the construction of 'who's-doing-whats' is an exercise in selection governed by social conventions and ideological systems.

The resources a language makes available for constructing 'who's-doing-whats' are part of the language's system of *transitivity*. This system provides different ways to represent 'doings' and the relationships between the participants (objects, people, places, practices) involved in them. 'Doings' (or 'processes'), may involve physical actions (material processes), mental actions (mental processes), communicative actions (verbal processes), the bodily display of thoughts and intentions (behavioral processes), and the demonstration of the relationships between things (relational processes). Participants may be linked together by these processes in different kinds of relationships with each other: They may be represented, for example, as *agents* performing a process on or to some other participant, as *patients*, having the process performed on or to them, or as benefactors, having the processes performed for them.

In texts having to do with health and risk this often results in the portrayal of social actors as having different degrees of agency over their health and health-related behavior. One good example of this is Francis and Kramer-Dahl's (1992) study of grammaticalization in medical case histories. Comparing a neurological case history published in an academic journal to a more popular account given in Oliver Sacks' *The Man who Mistook his Wife for a Hat* (1985), they observe that in the academic case history the patient is most often placed in what Hasan (1985) refers to as the '-ed role' or 'passive' role (for example: 'She was institutionalized because of poor memory' and 'She was discovered to have severe visual agnosia' (p. 60)). In other words, the patient is represented as essentially passive, being acted upon by (often unnamed) outside forces. This 'objectification' of the patient in the academic medical case history is contrasted with the way 'Dr P-', the patient in the title essay of Oliver Sacks' book is portrayed. Here, Francis and Kramer-Dahl note, the patient is more often placed in the '-er role', depicted as the 'doer' of actions. For example, he consults the doctor, observes and evaluates his own behavior, and is depicted as engaging in a whole range of activities such as dressing, singing, moving, and eating.

As I said above, like lexicalization, grammaticalization is fundamentally ideological, constructing certain kinds of people and promoting certain kinds of social practices. The grammatical choices observed here in neurological case histories are common to most written and verbal accounts of medical encounters from the perspective of the 'voice of medicine', in which doctors are usually portrayed as agents and patients are portrayed as 'patients' (in the grammatical sense). Sacks' grammatical choices, Francis and Kramer-Dahl argue, are designed not just as a challenge to the way medical case histories in neurology are written, but as a challenge to the way neurology itself is practiced and the asymmetrical power relations between doctors and patients that it entails.

The importance of agency in representations of health and risk can also be seen in health promotion discourse, the goal of which is usually to explain to people what to do in order to stay well and what not to do in order to avoid disease. The representation of agency in such texts can have an impact on what health promoters call 'self efficacy' (Bandura, 1990) – the degree to which texts amplify readers' sense of their own ability to take action to stay healthy or prevent disease.

An example of how health promotion discourse constructs social practices and social identities can be seen in my own study of AIDS prevention pamphlets produced in the People's Republic and China in the late 1990s (Jones, 2002a). In a corpus of fifty of these pamphlets I noted that human actors (including the readers of the pamphlets) are seldom depicted as agents in material processes. In other words, human actors are rarely portrayed as performing actions like 'using condoms' and 'not sharing needles'. Instead, the majority of material processes in the pamphlets are associated with inanimate objects, most commonly AIDS itself and the 'AIDS virus' (HIV), which is depicted as '*invading* the body', '*spreading* through the country', and '*destroying* the immune system'. This is not to say that human actors are never portrayed as agents in these texts. When they are, however, they are usually performing *mental processes* rather than material processes. Readers are advised to '*understand* AIDS', '*think about* their health, future and life', '*think about* their families', '*pay attention* to the fact that condoms are not 100% effective', '*remember* to be healthy and not to be promiscuous', and '*strengthen* self-protective *consciousness*'.

Just as 'correct' thought processes are represented as the primary means to avoid HIV infection, 'incorrect' thought processes are portrayed as the leading source of risk. An example of this can be seen in the story below from a booklet called *AIDS: The Warning of the Century* (Ceng and Ren, 1997, p. 43):

Wallowing in Degeneration

A young woman in a certain big city in China admired and yearned after a luxurious life. In order to satisfy her desires, she 'made friends' far and wide – no matter whether they were Chinese or foreigners, black or white – in an attempt to obtain money and beautiful clothes. She not only had no knowledge about AIDS, but also did not know that she herself had contracted the AIDS virus, and only blindly pursued her dream of marrying a foreigner and leaving the country. While she was living together with a Hong Kong businessman and preparing to get married, this couple both tested positive for the AIDS virus. Not long afterwards, the young woman developed full-blown AIDS and died far from home.

Here HIV infection is portrayed primarily as a consequence of mental processes. The character's downfall into 'degeneration', disease, and death is driven by 'admiring', 'yearning', 'blindly pursuing a dream', and 'not having knowledge about AIDS'. These mental processes are what cause the material processes such as 'making friends' with the wrong sorts of people. All of these mental processes converge in a 'state of consciousness' summed up with the four-character expression 'wallowing in degeneration' (自甘堕落) which forms the story's title.

In these materials, then, HIV transmission is constructed not so much as a matter of what people *do*, but of what they *think*, and protecting oneself against infection is the result of having certain kinds of thoughts and desires and avoiding other kinds. This reflects a broader 'moral model' of health promotion that dominated China during the time when these pamphlets were produced and to some extent persists today. This 'moral model' of health promotion, of course, is not unique to China or HIV, but can be seen in many cultural contexts, not only when it comes to issues like drug abuse and sexually transmitted diseases, but even when it comes to things like diet and exercise (Brandt and Rozin, 1997; Petersen and Lupton, 1996).

Nominalization

One of the chief ways grammaticalization contributes to the technologization of social practices is through the process of nominalization, the resource in language for turning processes into participants. As Hodge and Louie (1998, p. 84) describe it:

> This transformation takes a process involving actions and verbs, and turns it into a noun, a thing. In this form it loses many of its features as an action or process, and instead is fitted into a relational model where it becomes subordinated to processes of classification and judgment.

A number of scholars including Halliday and Martin (1993), Kress (1989), and Lemke (1990) have observed the tendency for scientific discourse (including medical discourse) to treat complex actions and activities as things that can be classified and evaluated. It also is a practice that Francis and Kramer-Dahl observe in the academic medical case histories they analyze, in which processes involving the patient are often encoded as nouns rather than as verbs in clauses such as: 'Auditory association learning was also very poor' (p. 64). Nominalization has the effect of making processes seem more 'solid', as well as more 'portable' – able to be separated from the specific circumstances in which they occurred and recontextualized into other circumstances. The following sentence from a paper in a medical journal, for example, contains a string of nominalized processes joined together in various relationships of co-temporality and cause and effect.

> Continuous intra-arterial pressure monitoring allowed rapid correction of any hypotension occurring during institution of anesthesia, or resulting from intraoperative blood loss.
>
> *(Brighouse and Guard, 1992, p. 519)*

What's striking about this example, though not at all unusual in biomedical discourse, is that the agents of these processes are invisible. There is no person monitoring the intra-arterial pressure, no person instituting the anesthesia or responsible for intraoperative blood loss. There are, of course, affordances for science in this way of describing phenomena. It gives writers a more efficient way to describe complex processes and make experiments or medical procedures more generalizable and easier to reproduce. In other words, it is the very power of nominalization to render actions decontextualizable, and thus to transform local phenomena into more distal 'facts' (Iedema, 2003a, 2003b) that makes it such an efficient tool for science and such an efficient means in general for the technologization of social practices.

It is also one of the features that make scientific discourse so opaque to many laypeople without the knowledge or experience needed to 'unpack' complex nominalizations. Thus, when doctors and scientists use nominalizations, the effect is sometimes to distance themselves from laypeople. In the BBC *Horizon* episode 'Does the MMR Jab Cause Autism?', many of the statements by 'experts' are heavy with nominalizations. Statistician Stephen Senn, for example, explains:

> I think that there's an inevitable tendency to mistake subsequence for con-sequence, that is to assume that because one particular event follows another, that therefore the preceding event caused it.

In this example, the first clause is dense with nominalizations in which complex processes are packed into words like 'tendency', 'subsequence', and 'consequence'. Although the second clause of the sentence attempts to 'unpack' these words, one wonders why the statistician did not use this simpler version in the first place, given that the program is intended for a general audience. This type of language contrasts dramatically with statements by parents on the program who vividly describe their autistic children's behavior in terms of concrete actions and events. In the following excerpt, for example, mother Rosemary Kessick demonstrates in her story the very 'inevitable tendency' Dr Senn deplores, but does so in language that is far more compelling to the average viewer:

> When William was born, he was wonderful. I had a great pregnancy, no problems at all. William was thriving and growing and jolly and bouncy and beautiful. William had an MMR at fifteen months and from then on he, for want of a better word, he disintegrated.

Nominalization, however, is not just a common tool in medical and scientific discourse; it also frequently appears in journalistic discourse in which complex (and often contested) phenomena and events are sometimes reduced to pat phrases. At the height of concerns about the safety of the MMR vaccine in Britain, for example, a story in the *Daily Mail* (February 2, 2002, cited in Speers and Lewis, 2004, p. 174) stated:

> Although health chiefs insist that the MMR vaccine is safe, many parents have been put off by *uncertainty* over possible *links* to autism and bowel disorders [emphasis mine].

What is interesting about this sentence is that it demonstrates how nominalizations, even when couched in the language of uncertainty, can sometimes make things seem more solidly established than they are. Two complex processes are nominalized here. One is the *linking* of autism to bowel disorders by Wakefield and his colleagues, which, although modalized ('possible'), is presented as much more certain than it actually was. The second thing that is nominalized is the process of public debate brought about by Wakefield's claims, glossed as *uncertainty*. As I mentioned above, one characteristic of nominalizations is that they sometimes erase participants and circumstances, allowing processes to 'float free'. Here it is unclear who is 'doing' the uncertainty – the parents, health chiefs, or scientists – and what the subject of this uncertainty is – the validity of links between the vaccine and autism or the safety of the vaccine itself.

The functions of nominalization in news discourse are in many ways not that different from its functions in scientific discourse: facilitating economy of expression, presenting certain information as background or 'given', and objectifying and depersonalizing information so that it can be more easily lifted out of specific situations and applied more generally. Just as the power of nominalization to construct 'free floating' practices helps to construct communities of doctors and research scientists who share common understandings of these practices, nominalization in news discourse helps to create communities of news readers who share understandings of certain events and phenomena.

Personalization

Personalization is the way that a text creates a relationship with a reader or viewer, constructing him or her as a certain kind of person. In texts concerned with health, personalization can have a considerable effect on how the meanings represented are taken up and used. Consider the following excerpt from the American Medical Association's *Guide to Talking to Your Doctor*.

> The lifestyle choices you make today will have a strong impact on your health in the future. Making the right choices now can help keep you healthy, while making the wrong choices can put your health at risk and even threaten your life. A number of diseases and conditions can be traced directly to risky behavior throughout a person's lifetime. These behaviors include eating a poor diet, exercising too little, smoking, abusing alcohol or other drugs, or having unsafe sex. Avoiding risky behaviors and living a healthier lifestyle are easy ways to prevent many diseases, injuries, and disabilities.
>
> *(American Medical Association, 2001, p. 33)*

In the first half of the paragraph, the writer speaks directly to the reader, addressing him or her as 'you' and using a conversational style, a common technique in persuasive discourse and particularly evident in many forms of health promotion. What the use of 'you' does in this passage is 'synthetically' (Fairclough, 1992a) construct an intimate relationship between the reader and the writer. It also creates a relationship between the reader and the content of the text, in this case making the reader solely responsible for various choices about his or her health. In the second half of the paragraph, however, a subtle shift in the relationship between the reader and the behavior under discussion occurs, with the 'you' of the first part of the passage disappearing. Rather than being associated with 'you', behaviors like 'eating a poor diet, exercising too little, smoking, abusing alcohol or other drugs, or having unsafe sex' are attributed to 'a person'. While the reader ('you') is portrayed as a 'choice maker' (who presumably 'makes the right choices'), it is others that are presented as 'risk takers', engaging in practices like 'abusing alcohol' and having 'unsafe sex'. There may be many reasons for this shift. It might be a way for the writer to avoid threatening the reader's face by imputing to him or her potentially socially unacceptable behaviors. It might also be a way of marginalizing those behaviors themselves (and the people who engage in them) by placing them outside the intimate sphere of the reader and the writer. The reading position made available by this text, however, does not take into account readers for whom avoiding these behaviors is *not* 'easy', whose 'poor diet', for example, might be a consequence of poverty or whose unsafe sex might be a result of being in an abusive relationship. In other words, not every reader is equally able to assume the identity this text makes available, even though this identity is presented as unproblematically universal.

The fact that texts construct their readers by making certain assumptions about them is an issue taken up by Hobson-West (2003) in her analysis of the NHS campaign to defuse the controversy surrounding MMR by presenting the public with 'the facts'. This strategy, Hobson-West argues, rests on the assumption that parents' decisions not to immunize their children are the result of a 'miscalculation of risk', and that the way to best solve the problem is to provide more accurate numerical information. In other words, by presenting 'the facts', the campaign constructs readers as ignorant of the facts. Many of these parents, however, may have come to their decision not on the basis of 'faulty calculations' but on the basis of the 'real-life' experiences of friends or people they had heard about, and giving them more 'facts' runs the risk of reinforcing their impression of public health officials as not respecting those 'real-life' experiences.

Mood

Personalization is chiefly accomplished through what Halliday (1973) calls the *interpersonal* resources for meaning available in a language, which include *mood* and *modality*. Mood refers to the resources a language makes available for constructing various 'discourse positions' (Kress, 1989) for producers and consumers of texts. Through different choices of mood (for example, declarative, imperative, or interrogative), texts designate to producers and consumers certain roles in the discourse (for example that of 'questioner' or 'answerer'), which, in different circumstances sometimes invoke larger social identities (for example those of teacher, student, doctor or patient) and the social practices associated with these identities.

Particularly important in texts about health and risk is the way mood selection contributes to a sense of involvement with or detachment from texts and their content (Hasan, 1985, p. 41). Francis and Kramer-Dahl (1992) illustrate this point in their comparison of mood structures in a traditional neurological case report and the more literary depiction by Oliver Sacks. In the traditional case report, nearly all of the clauses are declarative, constructing the author as 'an expert physician with his patient and expert writer with his readers' (p. 78). The declarative mood presents information in an objective way, opening up very little room for reader involvement. The writer/reader relationship is essentially asymmetrical, with the writer imparting information. The text by Sacks, on the other hand, includes not just declarative clauses but also a large number of imperative and especially interrogative clauses, mood types which are more likely to create in the reader a feeling of involvement with the text. Francis and Kramer-Dahl argue that through his frequent use of interrogatives, Sacks projects the image of a physician involved in a process of testing and revising his hypotheses, and by making this thought process visible in the text, he creates a more egalitarian relationship with his readers.

The issue of reader involvement associated with mood is, of course, of special importance in the discourse of health promotion, in which the degree of identification readers feel with the writers of texts can have an effect on their willingness to take up the messages in those texts. Like the text by Sacks discussed above, health promotion pamphlets and websites also make frequent use of the imperative and interrogative moods. The use of these moods, however, does not always result in the 'flattening' of hierarchies between reader and writer that Francis and Kramer-Dahl observe in the Sacks text. In fact, often these devices end up strengthening the hierarchical relationship between reader and writer. Imperatives, such as those found in the Chinese AIDS prevention pamphlets I analyzed like 'Don't give into the temptations of sexual liberation' and 'Don't let AIDS invade our beautiful country' obviously create an unequal relationship between the reader and the writer, who is constructed in this case as representing not just a moral authority but also a political one.

The interrogative mood can also contribute to the construction of asymmetrical relationships. Although it might seem an odd choice for a genre whose purpose is essentially to tell people what to do, interrogative constructions are particularly common in health promotion discourse, often appearing in lists of 'frequently asked questions' followed by their answers. Wright (1999) has noted that the use of the question/answer format in such materials makes them more 'reader friendly', helping busy people locate useful information by scanning the texts for questions that are relevant to their concerns. Another important effect of such questions, however, is to construct a certain kind of reader – a 'questioner' who lacks crucial knowledge and must depend upon experts to provide it. This technique not only makes assumptions about the kinds of things readers are ignorant or misinformed about, but also about the kinds of things they *ought* to know.

One possible consequence of this technique is to marginalize readers who feel they already have answers to the questions being asked (answers which are sometimes different from those given by the experts), along with those who might have different questions. Furthermore, the way authors of texts select and arrange questions and answers is not always ideologically neutral. This is particularly evident in the commercial brand of 'health promotion' engaged in by pharmaceutical companies. Johnson and Johnson's website for Extra Strength Tylenol (McNeil-PPC, 2011), for example, presents eighteen 'Frequently Asked Questions' about the product. The questions, however, are ordered in such a way that those closer to the top of the list are of an essentially promotional nature, focusing on the positive attributes of the product, questions like: 'What are the advantages of TYLENOL®?' It is not until the bottom of the list that the reader comes across the arguably more important questions about the product's safety such as 'Does TYLENOL® cause liver damage?'

Modality

Another important grammatical resource used in the process of personalization is the language's system of modality, the system through which things like certainty and obligation are expressed. Modality also has a particular importance in discourse around health and risk given that two central functions of such discourse are to discuss the probability that certain behaviors will result in certain diseases or medical conditions and to communicate to people what they should or should not do to avoid these diseases or medical conditions. Modality is usually expressed through the use of *modal verbs* (such as can, may, might) and *modal adjuncts* (such as probably, usually, evidently, generally, unfortunately). Although they are usually associated with the ideational function of language, *circumstantial adjuncts*, especially in the form of casual or conditional expressions, also play a major role in communicating about risk and uncertainty in health-related discourse.

In the answer to the question 'Does TYLENOL® cause liver damage?' on the Tylenol website, for example, the authors write:

> When taken as directed, according to the package label, TYLENOL® (acetaminophen) does not cause liver damage.
> In situations where an excessive amount of acetaminophen has been ingested, such as in the case of an overdose, liver damage may occur.

The first thing to notice about this answer is that there are actually two answers associated with two different kinds of circumstances ('When taken as directed … ' and 'In situations where an excessive amount of acetaminophen has been ingested'). The degree of certainty assigned to the risk under the first condition is categorical (TYLENOL® *does not cause liver damage*), whereas under the second condition, the degree of certainty is qualified by the use of a modal verb (liver damage *may* occur). The obvious effect of these choices is to downplay the degree of risk associated with the product.

There are aspects of this text apart from modality, however, which also contribute to the downplaying of the risk of liver damage associated with Tylenol. One has to do with the ordering of the clauses. By choosing to 'thematize' the circumstantial adjuncts (that is, put them at the beginning of the sentences) – a choice that in English is considered marked – the author further emphasizes the conditionality of the risk. There is, as well, a clear difference in the style or 'social language' in which the first and the second sentences are written. The first sentence is written in a simple and direct style which uses common vocabulary and active voice (TYLENOL® does not cause liver damage), whereas the second sentence is written in more complex 'scientific language' with a long circumstantial adjunct containing more specialized vocabulary ('excessive', 'ingested') and a passive construction which avoids explicitly assigning agency to TYLENOL®. Finally, it is also important to notice that in the second sentence the product is referred to by its generic name – the brand name is not mentioned. The effect of these choices becomes dramatically clear if we simply switch the information in the two sentences to read:

> In situations where an appropriate amount of acetaminophen has been ingested, liver damage may not occur.
>
> When too much is taken, TYLENOL® (acetaminophen) does cause liver damage.

Organization

By organization I mean the way texts are structured and sequenced, and how meanings are linked together. Here, however, I am interested not just in those features in texts that create cohesion and coherence, what Halliday calls the 'textual' metafunction, but more importantly in how the conventional structures that texts follow function to organize social practices and social identities, social relationships, and social groups (Iedema, 2003a).

Texts are constructed according to sets of expectations within particular communities about how texts of a certain sort should be constructed. These expectations have to do with things like the order of information in the text, the style in which the text is written, and the inclusion of various modes like graphics. Many health-related genres (including health promotion pamphlets like those I considered above), for example, follow a classic 'problem-solution structure' (Hoey, 1994), in which the presentation of a problem is followed by the presentation of a solution. This structure is also exploited by advertisements for health products such as over-the-counter medications. In fact, pharmaceutical companies refer to this as the 'lock and key' structure, in which the drug is portrayed as the solution (key) to open the 'lock' of a particular disease (Parry, 2003).

Narratives of various kinds also play an important role in discourse about health and risk (see chapter 6). One example is the ritualistic 'recovery story' prevalent in 'twelve-step' programs like Alcoholics Anonymous, which typically begins with 'the first drink' and follows a narrative of denial and decline to a moment of 'hitting bottom', an admission of 'powerlessness', and an acceptance of a 'higher power' (Jones, 2005a). This narrative formula has its antecedents in confessional genres that date back to the Middle Ages, but the modern template is the story of 'Bill W.'

as told in the book *Alcoholics Anonymous* (known as the 'Big Book'). A big part of being socialized into these programs involves learning how to competently reproduce this schematic structure. For members socialized into these communities, what is important about these formulaic stories is not so much the details of the individual teller's experiences, but the way the *structure* of the story links their experiences to those of others in the group (Jensen, 2000; Jones, 2005a).

The way readers draw upon templates or organizational 'schemata' when interacting with texts has long been a concern of applied linguists and others interested in text comprehension (see for example Rumelhart, 1975; Schank and Abelson, 1977; Tannen, 1993; van Dijk, 2008). Such schemata link texts both to individual processes of cognition and to the social practices of communities, institutions, and cultures: text structures help members of communities coordinate their actions and create a sense of shared experience. People from different communities, in fact, might 'read into' the same texts different principles of organization.

An example of this can be seen in a study I undertook in the mid-1990s which compared the ways Chinese students in Hong Kong interpreted televised AIDS prevention messages to the way the same messages were interpreted by their British and American lecturers (Jones, 1996). Participants in the study were shown identical versions of Hong Kong Government AIDS awareness commercials in Cantonese and English and asked to 'retell' them. The Chinese students mostly structured their responses as narratives. They interpreted the commercials as 'moral stories' in which HIV infection was the consequence of the characters' actions. Expatriate viewers, on the other hand, tended to see the commercials in more abstract, analytical terms, talking about the 'messages' they were trying to convey or technical aspects like cinematography.

There are many reasons why the Chinese students in this study might have been more likely to regard these commercials as 'moral stories' and the expatriates were more likely to regard them as 'lectures'. Kleinman (1980), for example, has pointed out the moral dimension of disease in Chinese societies, and others (see for example Fung, 1994; Metzger, 1981) have observed how narratives tend to play a didactic role in the socialization of Chinese children. Many of the AIDS prevention pamphlets from China I discussed above also present explicitly moral messages, often in the form of stories. Studies of audience reactions to health promotion in Northern Europe and the United States (see for example Baggaley, 1993), on the other hand, show a preference for an anti-rhetorical, 'facts based' approach.

I do not, however, wish here to propose any blanket statements about how 'Chinese culture' or 'Western culture' affects the way people interpret messages about health and risk (see chapter 8). Indeed, the different responses of the different groups in this study might have had just as much to do with the fact that they were 'students' and 'lecturers'. What I would like to point out, though, is that different people bring to texts about health and risk different expectations about organization, which can have an effect on how they interpret messages.

The ways texts are organized does not just reflect the cognitive schemata and shared interpretative repertoires of people of different communities. It also makes possible many of the activities that bind those communities together. In other words, attention to the process of organization is not just about how texts are organized, but also about how the organization of texts functions to organize people and their social practices (see chapter 8). Yanoff (1988), for example, has identified the six key professional genres in medicine and linked them with the kinds of professional roles physicians engage in when they use them. They are case write-ups (for medical students), discharge summaries (for house officers), consultation letters and case reports (for private practitioners), and published reports of original research and grant proposals (for academic physicians). Demonstrating competence in these genres through professional 'rituals' like the oral presentation of case reports for medical students and the peer review of proposals for academic physicians is an important part of enacting these roles.

Resemiotization

The final process I will discuss is particularly important because it to some degree determines how all of the other processes are carried out: it involves the choice of the semiotic modes and the materialities through which knowledge, experience, and relationships are entextualized. As I mentioned at the start of this chapter, all acts of entextualization involve the creation of more or less durable *artifacts* out of dynamic and transient phenomena. Biological processes are transformed into diagnoses. Experiences stretching over days or weeks or years are transformed into narratives. Clinical trials are turned into scientific papers, and later into recommendations by scientific or government bodies, and finally into pamphlets recommending certain treatments or health behaviors.

Different semiotic modes (such as language, numbers, pictures) and different materialities (printed texts, digital documents, video or audio recordings) all have different affordances and constraints in terms of which aspects of reality they are able to represent and which they are not. Numbers, for example, can express exact amounts, but depend upon readers for interpretation, whereas verbal expressions of quantification (many, some, a few) interpret and add 'values' to quantities, though they are unable to express the same degree of exactness. A chest X-ray can express the state of affairs in a patient's lungs at a particular moment, but cannot tell us how the lungs ended up in that state in the way a patient's narrative or medical history might be able to. And a note scribbled on a patient's chart indicating the presence of lymphadenopathy cannot fully capture the fine gradations of swelling detected by the palpitating fingers of a doctor. Because of these differences in affordances between modes, when we translate meanings, experiences, and relationships from one mode to another, we always end up changing them in some way, highlighting certain aspects of them and obscuring others.

One of the most important differences in terms of the affordances and constraints of different modes is that, as Kress and van Leeuwen (1996) have pointed out, some modes like language operate according to the logic of time, with one thing coming after another in a way that the order of information can be very important

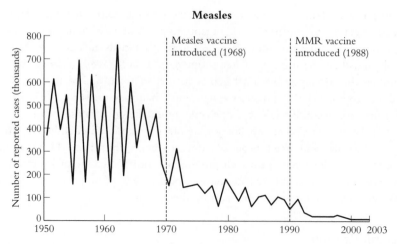

FIGURE 3.1 Measles, from *MMR: The Facts* (NHS, 2004)

for the message, whereas other modes like images operate according to a spatial logic which allows readers to take in information in a way that depends less upon sequential ordering. This is one reason why graphs like that in Figure 3.1 showing the number of reported cases of measles in Britain over a 53-year period published in *MMR: The Facts* is in many ways a more dramatic presentation of the vaccine's effectiveness than a verbal account or a table because it allows readers to 'see' the high rates of measles in the 1950s and 1960s and the low rates in the 1990s at the same time, moving their eyes back and forth to compare them.

Another reason such representations are particularly effective is that they allow readers to also 'see' the slope of the decrease in a way that language can only portray with less exact words like 'steep' and 'gradual'. As Lemke (1998) points out, language favors *typological* meaning-making, the division of phenomena into 'types' (colors, sizes, symptoms, and diseases), whereas visual modes allow for more *topological* meaning-making in which fine gradations of things like color, size, swelling, and slope can be expressed. Of course graphs like the one pictured in Figure 3.1 are not truly topological in the way photographs can be – the line actually connects up a number of discrete data points rather than showing a continuous ebb and flow of cases. Nevertheless, presenting these separate data points in this way gives the impression of topological meaning, an impression that can sometimes be deceptive depending on the way the data points are spread out and what was actually happening between them.

Different topics and purposes for communication, of course, tend to call for more typological or more topological meaning-making. One domain of communication in which the limits of typological meaning-making are particularly evident is communication about pain, and the following text (Figure 3.2) is an example of one way these limitations can be addressed by offering readers multiple modes through which to conceptualize and communicate pain.

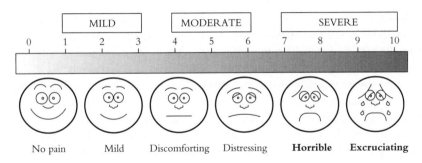

FIGURE 3.2 Pain Management Scale

This text makes available to users five different ways to communicate about the intensity of pain, some more typological and some more topological. The verbal expressions of intensity are examples of typological meaning: pain is expressed in terms of different 'kinds' of intensity, on the top of the chart from an 'objective', 'relative' point of view, reflecting the perspective (and the register) of the doctor ('MILD', 'MODERATE' and 'SEVERE'), and, on the bottom of the chart, from the more subjective point of view of the patient ('Discomforting', 'Distressing', 'Horrible'). The words at the bottom of the chart also make use of the font as a resource for meaning, with 'Horrible' and 'Excruciating' appearing in bold type. The band of color in the center of the chart, on the other hand, in which pain is metaphorically represented as being related to colors (from 'cool' blues to 'intense' oranges and reds) is an example of topological meaning, each color blending into the next along the continuum of the spectrum. The numbers on top of the band of color and the faces below it represent modes that combine both typological and topological meaning-making. The numbers 0 to 10 spaced evenly along a 100 mm horizontal line are a widely used tool for measuring pain in medicine known as the visual analog scale (Aitken, 1969). It is typological in that it presents a set of discrete points of reference, each representing a different intensity, but at the same time typological in that these points are placed at equal intervals along a continuous line along which patients can place their pain, regardless of whether it falls on one of the points of reference or somewhere between two of them. The set of faces, another widely used measurement tool known as the Wong-Baker FACES Pain Rating Scale (Wong and Baker, 1988) also to some degree combines both kinds of meaning: although only six faces are presented, each representing a discrete expression, the images are based on a system of meaning-making (facial expressions) that is itself topological.

The important point about the combination of these modes in this text, how-ever, is not how they operate separately, but how they interact with one another. In fact, the whole point of this text is to facilitate the 'translation' of one kind of meaning-making into another – to help patients transform their more subjective, topological experience of pain into the more abstract, typological language of doctors.

Another important aspect of resemiotization is the materiality of the media in which experiences are entextualized. As I mentioned above, one of the primary ways the act of entextualization contributes to the technologization of social practices and social identities is through instantiating them in progressively 'solid' forms. The momentary words, gestures, and physical contact of a medical examination are transformed into a more durable written record, which then might be transformed into a concrete treatment involving drugs or surgery which alters the physical body of the patient. A conversation between a husband and wife about strategies to lower their cholesterol leads to the collection of texts like recipes and exercise programs, which are further transformed into meals and 5 km runs in the wooded areas around their home. As I said in the last chapter, one of the goals of an applied linguistic approach to health and risk communication should be to follow the itineraries along which discourse travels as it is transformed from talk, to written texts, to actions, and back into talk. These moments of resemiotization and rematerialization, I argued, are key to understanding the relationship between discourse and the concrete actions we take around health and risk.

*

I began this chapter by discussing the differences between narrative and analytical ways of organizing knowledge and social relationships around health and how these different organizational principles amplify and constrain different kinds of responses to health issues and serve to align producers and consumers of texts to different communities (doctors, scientists, journalists, and 'parents'). I then went on to show how different ways of representing health and risk go beyond these broad principles of organization to include the kinds of words we use, the ways we represent actions and states of being and assign agency to social actors, the way we construct relationships between readers and writers and express things like certainty and obligation, the way we build texts around cognitive schemata and community practices, and the modes and materialities through which we communicate. One important point that has arisen from this discussion is that meanings do not reside solely in texts. Rather, texts form an interface between individual cognition and social groups and their practices. What determines the way different experiences and relationships get entextualized is not just the fact that different people and different groups have access to different kinds of knowledge, but also that they have access to different *strategies of knowledge management* (van Dijk, 2003).

Understanding the ways social practices and social identities are technologized in texts, however, is only part of understanding the relationship between discourse and health. Another important aspect, which I will consider in the next two chapters, is how people negotiate these practices and identities in situated social interactions like medical consultations, conversations with friends, interactions around dinner tables, and sexual encounters.

4

SITES OF ENGAGEMENT

In the last chapter I considered the role of texts in helping to 'technologize' social practices and social identities around health and risk. In this chapter I will focus on the *sites of engagement* (Jones, 2005c; Scollon, 2001a) into which these social practices and social identities are appropriated to take concrete, real-time actions. A site of engagement is a moment when particular kinds of people and particular 'cultural tools' come together to make certain kinds of social actions possible. Sites of engagement are not static 'contexts' in which interaction takes place. They are actively constructed moment by moment by participants as they make use of the texts and other tools that are available to them.

Much of what occurs at sites of engagement is determined by the 'technologized' social practices and social identities that we bring to them. People who enter doctors' offices do so with a pretty good idea about the sorts of social practices that will occur in them, the sorts of texts they will be required to produce and consume, and the sorts of social identities they will be expected to assume. At the same time, every medical encounter is different, and doctors and patients must be prepared to engage in different kinds of practices and assume different kinds of identities as contingencies change. All sites of engagement have these two dimensions: they are, as Sarangi and Roberts (1999, p. 18) put it, both 'brought along' – determined by the social practices and social identities that people bring to them – and 'brought about' through the strategic ways people use language and other tools to *perform* social practices and *enact* social identities in real time.

All sites of engagement depend upon how participants accomplish the two basic tasks of negotiating 'what they are doing' and 'who they are being' (Scollon, 1998). I will be referring to the ways in which people strategically manage social practices and social identities in their interactions as 'framing' and 'positioning'. 'Framing' refers to the metacommunicative management of *social practices* in interaction, and positioning refers to the metacommunicative management of *social identities*. It is through these two processes that participants in encounters open 'windows of opportunity' that make particular kinds of actions and relationships possible (Scollon, 2001b).

Opening these windows of opportunity is not always easy. There are situations in which, for any number of reasons, the expectations that different people bring to the interaction about what they should be doing and who they should be being are different, due to their access to different repertoires of social practices and social identities. There are also situations in which participants put forth framings and positionings that are at odds with each other because of different goals or agendas. Finally, there are sites of engagement which are themselves ambiguous – sites like genetic counseling sessions (Sarangi, 2000), commercial sex encounters (Jones, 2002a, 2007), and health promotion events in public places (Jones, 2002b) in which multiple 'activity types' (Levinson, 1979; Sarangi, 2000) and social identities mix in rather complex ways.

I know this from personal experience in my capacity as a volunteer for an AIDS service organization in Hong Kong. Every year on World AIDS Day the organization I belong to gets its volunteers to hand out AIDS prevention information and condoms to people on the streets. Sometimes on these occasions my social identity is an issue, with passersby who are not familiar with the practice looking quizzical when I hand them a condom. The social identities of the recipients of these items are also an issue. When handing out condoms, for example, certain passersby (children, Buddhist monks) are intentionally overlooked. This became problematic one year when our organization decided to package the condoms in red envelopes of the kind used during Chinese New Year to give 'lucky money' to children. On this occasion small children took to following me with outstretched hands, requiring me to explain to their angry parents why I was withholding these 'red packets' from their sons and daughters.

Applied linguists have dealt with the dual problems of framing and positioning using a variety of analytical frameworks, and the fact that the terms I am using are associated with 'interactional sociolinguistics' should not be taken to limit their definitions to those narrowly associated with this approach. Rather, I mean the terms to apply broadly to the processes by which people in interaction negotiate their activities and their identities at multiple levels. The way activities are framed, for example, might be seen in the rather broad terms favored by ethnographers of communication to mean the sets of fundamental assumptions that govern how different kinds of speech events should be structured. Or it might be seen in the narrower perspective of how people strategically 'bring about' activities in actual encounters, using a variety of 'contextualization cues' to negotiate 'what's going on'. Or, it might be seen from the micro-analytical perspective of conversation analysts for whom a single utterance creates the 'frame' for how the next utterance is to be interpreted. Similarly, the question of social identity can be approached on many levels: on the broader level of fixed social roles, as a more strategic matter of 'performance' (Goffman, 1959), as the discursive negotiation of relational issues like power and solidarity, and as the turn-by-turn procedures through which people in conversation make themselves 'recognizable' to each other.

As analysts we can approach interactions on any of these different levels. We might, for example, analyze a medical consultation as a 'structured event' and try to determine the kind of 'communicative competence' (Hymes, 1974) participants need to bring to it, or we can see it as an 'interactional stream' (ten Have, 1995, p. 253) in which practices and identities are locally negotiated through the accomplishment of sequential talk. In this chapter I will, after Cicourel (1992), argue for a multi-dimensional approach to the issues of framing and positioning, one which takes into account both 'broad' and 'narrow' aspects of context (p. 292) and social identity and attempts to understand how they are related, how social and institutional orders construct and constrain the actions and identities people are able to perform at any given moment, and how the moment-by-moment negotiation of activities and identities acts to sustain (and sometimes to challenge) social and institutional orders (Sarangi and Roberts, 1999).

Most of the work in applied linguistics on health-related social interaction has taken place in clinical settings, and this chapter will focus primarily on such settings. At the same time, there is also a growing body of work on interactions that do not take place in clinics with healthcare professionals but rather involve the negotiation of health and risk in people's everyday lives. This will be the focus of the next chapter.

What are we doing?

The main problem with negotiating 'what we are doing' in interactions, whether they take place in consultation rooms or bedrooms, is that typically we are doing more than one thing at a time, and these different 'doings' are arranged in complex patterns of *sequentiality* and *simultaneity* in interactions. Participants in interactions must not only work to accomplish various actions at the 'right time' and in the 'right order', but they must also work to 'align' their actions with those of other participants.

A number of scholars have attributed difficulties in communication in clinical settings to a lack of alignment between healthcare workers and their patients regarding their understanding of 'what's going on' (see for example Chenail, 1991; Evans et al., 1986; Keeney, 1987). One reason for this is that doctors and patients 'bring along' to consultations different goals and expectations. Another reason, however, is that medical consultations themselves are complex activities in which, from the point of view of both the doctor and the patient, numerous things must 'get done', and managing shifts from one activity to another can sometimes be complicated.

Sequential frames

Medical consultations are typically carried out in stages in which each stage is devoted to the accomplishment of a particular task or set of tasks. Not only does the whole interaction involve certain expectations brought along by participants regarding the order in which the stages should be accomplished, but each stage or 'sequential frame' of the interaction has its own sets of expectations associated with it.

The classic formulation of the stages of the medical consultation comes from Byrne and Long (1976), who divide it into six stages:

1. relating to the patient
2. discovering the reason for attendance
3. conducting a verbal or physical examination or both
4. consideration of the patient's condition
5. detailing treatment or further investigation
6. terminating.

Later scholars, however, have criticized this model as focusing only on how the doctor frames 'what's going on' and ignoring the perspective of the patient. Ten Have (1989) consequently revised the sequence to be more participant neutral, labeling the six stages as follows:

1. opening
2. complaint
3. examination or test
4. diagnosis
5. treatment or advice
6. closing.

As I said above, each of these phases is devoted to a specific task or tasks which must to some extent be jointly accomplished by both patient and doctor, tasks such as complaint presentation, history-taking, advice-giving, and the writing of prescriptions (Heath, 1986). The sequence in which these phases occur, of course, is not arbitrary. Not only is the order of the sequence determined by a relationship of 'conditional relevance' (Schegloff, 1968) between phases, with one phase creating the necessary conditions for the next phase to occur, but there is also a certain 'momentum' associated with these phases so that it becomes difficult sometimes to return to previous phases once new phases have been initiated: it is difficult, for example, for patients to revise their complaints after a treatment has been prescribed (though this sometimes happens).

Each of these phases also has its own typical set of discourse characteristics and its own set of conversational actions (or 'moves') that are also sequentially organized (ten Have, 1991). These more locally organized actions (such as question–answer sequences) both contribute to the accomplishment of different phases and are themselves framed by the phases in which they occur, so that a question might accomplish something very different in the complaint phase than in the treatment phase.

Different scholars have focused on describing the characteristics of these different phases, Beckman and Frankel (1984) and Marvel and her colleagues (1999), for example, concentrating on the 'complaint' frame, Ainsworth-Vaughn (1998) and Maynard (1991) focusing on diagnosis, and Roberts (1999) focusing on treatment recommendations. What they have found is that certain sequential frames are more likely to accommodate certain types of discourse. For example, Chatwin (2006) observes that narratives from patients are much less likely to be attenuated or interrupted by physicians when they come in the initial presenting-complaint and history-taking segment of the examination when the doctor is most able to listen to what the patient is saying. Heritage and Stivers (1999, p. 1501) have noted that the examination phase is often accompanied by a unique type of talk they call the 'online commentary', 'talk that describes what the physician is seeing, feeling or hearing' (see also Mangione-Smith, Stivers, Elliott, McDonald, and Heritage, 2003). And Mitchum (1989) has pointed out that the diagnosis phase, likely as it is to involve more technical language, usually includes more explanation on the part of the doctor, though others (see for example Ainsworth-Vaughn, 1998) have pointed out that physicians sometimes limit patients' ability to ask questions or issue challenges during this stage.

It should be clear from the above observations that doctors (and sometimes patients as well) use sequential frames (and the discourse conventions that govern them) in various strategic ways, sometimes to facilitate the performance of particular tasks, and sometimes to avoid engaging in tasks they do not wish to engage in. Barton (2004), for example, shows how doctors in the oncology practice she observed regularly exploit the lack of a generic move for presenting a prognosis in the treatment stage of the consultation in order to avoid giving patients a prognosis altogether, thus sparing themselves the difficulties inherent in delivering bad news.

At the same time, many scholars have noted that actual interactions between doctors and patients are sometimes not as neat as this model implies. Sarangi (2010b), for example, shows how, in talk between doctors and patients' parents in pediatric encounters, episodes of examination and the discussions of symptoms and treatments often occur at multiple times throughout consultations in sequences that do not conform with the classic phases of the medical encounter. This is particularly true, he notes, in encounters where the goals of the doctor and the patient's parent are not aligned, as when the parent comes to the encounter seeking a prescription for antibiotics and the doctor does not regard the prescription as warranted. In such cases, deviation from the expected sequence can be seen as strategic, the doctor initiating recursive phases of examination and complaint-taking to delay the treatment phase. In contrast, he found that consultations in which doctors were willing to prescribe antibiotics tended to be shorter and follow a more conventional structure.

Other researchers have noted how particular phases in medical encounters are vulnerable to being 'contaminated' by activities that can hinder rather than facilitate the accomplishment of the phase. Ten Have (1989) discusses, for instance, how, especially in the complaint phase, patients can sometimes slip into the activity of 'troubles telling' (the elaboration of the trouble beyond what is 'technically necessary' for successful diagnosis) and doctors can sometimes slip into 'therapy talk' (encouraging the patient to engage in unnecessary self-reflection and refusing to give expert advice). The problem with both of these activities, of course, is that they often take longer than is usually possible in a typical medical consultation. He also notes how some patients exploit pauses in the consultation in order to add to their complaints or change their complaints altogether long after the complaint frame has been closed, even at the stage at which the physician is actually writing out the prescription. He calls the phenomenon of doctors and patients being 'out of phase' with each other 'interactional asynchrony'.

Despite these observations, many studies show that both doctors and patients actively work to avoid such asynchrony. Not only do doctors regularly interrupt patients when they feel things are getting 'off track' (Måseide, 1991) or encourage them to pursue one particular line of talk rather than another (Aronsson and Sätterlund-Larsson, 1987), but patients also regularly check that what they are saying is in alignment with the doctor's expectations by, for example, using upward 'questioning' intonation and pausing to let doctors issue confirmations of the 'doctorability' of what is being said (Chatwin, 2006, p. 118).

Most studies describing the delicate interactional work that doctors and patients engage in to manage the sequential phases of their encounters have focused on dyadic interactions where a single healthcare worker is dealing with a single patient. Issues of interactional asynchrony become much more complex in situations in which different healthcare workers may be involved in different stages of the consultation, as occurs in emergency department visits like those observed by Slade and her colleagues (2008). In such interactions, some of the stages such as history-taking and examination are typically repeated multiple times as the patient makes his or her journey through the emergency department. The multiple personnel involved in different stages and the frequent repetition of stages can sometimes leave patients confused about 'what's going on' and about where they are in the overall process.

Interactive frames

Within the broader sequential framing of activities there might also occur moments when physicians or patients are engaging in multiple, *simultaneous* activities for which they must negotiate *interactive frames* (Goffman, 1974; Tannen and Wallat, 1987). The classic description of this phenomenon in health communication is Tannen and Wallat's (1987) analysis of a pediatric consultation in which the doctor juggles the different tasks of examining an eight-year-old cerebral palsied child, explaining what is going on to the child's mother, and reporting on the procedure for medical residents who will later watch it on videotape. In the interaction the doctor uses a variety of strategies such as shifts in word choice, grammar, and prosody as well as non-verbal communication like facial expressions to signal the different frames of 'examining the child', 'explaining to the mother', and 'lecturing the residents'. In examining the child, for example, she uses a teasing register characterized by extreme shifts in pitch, drawn-out vowel sounds, and smiling. She also laminates the examination with a 'play frame', engaging the child in an elaborate game involving looking for animals and peanut butter and jelly sandwiches in various parts of her body. When reporting on the procedure for the residents, her tone is flat and marked by sophisticated medical terminology which neither the child nor the mother could be expected to understand. And when she speaks to the mother she uses a conventional conversational register. What is challenging about managing the framing of simultaneous activities is that different frames may involve ways of behaving that conflict with the demands of other frames. Answering a parent's questions, for example, might interfere with examining the child, and reporting findings to the video audience might entail the use of technical vocabulary, which may make necessary even more explanation to the parent.

Other researchers have also documented how healthcare workers and patients make strategic use of interactive frames in consultations. Beck and Ragan (1992), for example, show how nurse practitioners use subtle cues to shift between a medical examination frame and a relational 'small talk' frame as a way of dispelling the embarrassment associated with the examination, and Justine Coupland and her colleagues (1994) discuss how doctors and elderly patients work together to mix and blend socio-relational and medical frames in ways that help to make their encounters seem less clinical.

While the management of framing is difficult when participants are engaged in multiple activities at once, it can be even more problematic when the purpose of the encounter itself involves a certain amount of ambiguity and hybridity. Sarangi (2000) points out such ambiguity in genetic counseling encounters, which in some ways resemble traditional medical encounters where healthcare workers issue what amount to diagnoses and recommendations, and in other ways resemble therapeutic encounters in which clients are encouraged to come to their own conclusions and healthcare workers strive to be non-directive. Sarangi argues that genetic counseling is a hybrid activity type, and, in order to manage this hybridity, counselors must combine, adapt, and transform discourse types (Fairclough, 1992a) in strategic ways. One example is the way genetic counselors often deal with advice-seeking from clients by treating requests for advice as opportunities to offer further explanations, transforming 'advice-seeking moves' into 'information-as-explanation giving sequences' (Sarangi, 2000, p. 19).

The phenomenon of overlapping, interactive frames is particularly relevant to the kind of complex interactions in emergency rooms mentioned above, in which doctors, nurses, and medical technicians are often involved in multitasking, shifting back and forth from patient to patient and from activity to activity. In such situations, however, frame shifts may be governed more by contingency than strategy, and may sometimes result in confusion or difficulties in communication among members of medical teams. Iedema (2011) borrows from Pickering (1995) the term 'mangle of practice' to describe how in such sites of engagement practices, cultural tools, and human beings are 'mangled together' in unpredictable ways.

Temporal frames

Apart from the *sequential frames* that make up medical encounters, and the multiple simultaneous actions people must often manage in these encounters through *interactive frames*, interactions in clinics and hospitals can also be seen in terms of inter-nested *temporal frames* of discrete actions that go to make larger activities, which themselves are part of even longer-scale processes. A patient's visit to the doctor, for example, is always part of a longer experience with a particular set of symptoms; this bout of symptoms may be part of a longer disease trajectory; and the disease itself can be seen in terms of a lifetime history of health and illness. Similarly, from the doctor's point of view, the visit can be seen as part of a workday, which can be seen in terms of a work week, a stage in the doctor's professional development, and a longer medical career. And from the point of view of the institution, the visit can be seen in terms of broader administrative cycles of work schedules, record keeping, planning, and reporting. In other words, just as our analysis of the consultation can be 'scaled down' to examine discrete activities like 'history-taking', or to examine the fine details of the interaction like adjacency sequences and interruptions, so can our analysis be 'scaled up' to consider the longer-timescale activities of individuals and institutions of which the consultation forms a part.

Here Lemke's (2000) notion of 'timescales' is particularly useful. All interactions, he says, consist of multiple activities occurring on different timescales, with shorter timescale activities going to make longer timescale ones, and longer timescale activities imposing constraints on what can occur on shorter timescales. The key point that Lemke makes is not just that 'lower level actions' occur in the context of 'higher level actions' (Norris and Jones, 2005; Scollon, 2001a), but that how lower-level and higher-level actions turn out depends crucially on their relationship with one another. A doctor, for example, treats an episode of fainting differently if he or she sees it as part of a longer history of fainting spells than if it is regarded at the level of a single incident. Blommaert (2005) makes a similar point when he talks of the 'layered simultaneity' of discourse, the overlapping of different timescales from the slow-moving *longue durée* (long term) along which things like scientific discoveries and healthcare systems develop to the short-term trajectories of momentary encounters. It is important to remember, he reminds us, that actions on these different timescales do not necessarily develop coherently. 'Different aspects of reality', he writes, 'could develop at different speeds' (p. 128). This seems particularly evident in texts and conversations about health and risk in which the temporal frames within which threats are set can have a profound effect on people's perception of the magnitude of the threats. Chandran and Menton (2004) have found, for example, that when information on the prevalence of heart attacks is given in the framework of daily rather than yearly incidence, people are more likely to see the risk as more proximal and concrete and to take action to try to avoid it.

Some of the difficulties professionals and laypeople have in communicating about things like risks and treatments may come from the two parties approaching these issues through different temporal frameworks. For patients, for example, the short-term benefits of a particular behavior like drinking or smoking might seem more immediate than the long-term benefits of quitting, or, conversely, they may see long-term benefits to certain behaviors (like unprotected sex with a potential long-term partner), where physicians and counselors might focus more on the more immediate dangers (see chapter 5).

The way participants manage temporal framing is particularly important in contexts like genetic counseling where counselors and clients work together to interpret and reinterpret information within different timeframes sometimes stretching back to the distant past, other times extending into a distant and often uncertain future (Sarangi et al., 2004). Discursive acts of 'circumferencing' (Scollon and Scollon, 2004) can have the effect of reassuring clients or of instilling in them a sense of urgency, and genetic counselors use them strategically to help people make sense of information and make decisions about future actions. In fact, a genetic test itself is a particularly powerful semiotic artifact for mediating between timescales, making timescales of lifetimes and even generations relevant to the actions on shorter timescales.

Who are we being?

Just as interaction involves constantly negotiating 'what we are doing' against a backdrop of socially recognized and institutionally sanctioned social practices, it also involves an ongoing process of claiming and imputing identities for ourselves against a backdrop of recognized and institutionally sanctioned social identities. All activities around health, whether engaging in a potentially risky sexual interaction, delivering health promotion messages, or seeking treatment in a hospital emergency room, are always acts of identity, and, whether or not a sexual interaction is safe or risky, a health promotion message is accepted or rejected, or treatment progresses smoothly in an institutional setting depends on the moment-by-moment management of 'who we are being'.

In much sociological theory, especially from a functionalist perspective, the question of 'who we are being' in interactions is seen in terms of 'roles' that involve fairly stable sets of rights and obligations. In medical sociology the most famous articulation of this approach is Parson's (1951) formulation of 'the sick role'. Although widely criticized for being too static, the model of the 'sick role' does succeed in highlighting how interactions are often constrained by normative expectations about the kinds of behavior associated with different participants (Fahy and Smith, 1999). More interactionalist accounts of role, on the other hand, like those of Goffman (1959) and Mead (1934), focus more on the contingent and locally emergent nature of performances.

Others, when considering the question of 'who we are being' in interactions, speak in terms of 'identity'. 'Identity' is a notoriously ambiguous term, used to describe everything from the unique properties that distinguish one person from another to the social categories that we claim for ourselves or impose on others (Erickson, 1994; Tajfel and Turner, 1986). Brubaker and Cooper (2000) make the distinction between identity as a 'category of practice' – the way people make sense of their selves and activities in everyday life – and identity as a 'category of analysis' – the way social scientists make sense of people and their activities, and they warn of the dangers of confusing the two. The job of the analyst, they insist, is to neither adopt uncritically 'categories of practice' as 'categories of analysis', nor to dismiss them as entirely constructed and contingent, but rather to 'explain the processes and mechanisms through which ... "identity" can crystallize at certain moments as a powerful, compelling reality' (p. 5).

This is, in fact, the point of view adopted by most applied linguists, for whom identity is seen both as something that is performed as people expose various aspects of themselves at different moments in interaction (F. Erickson, 1996; Schiffrin, 1996), and as something that is negotiated with other people through the discursive invocation of mutually recognizable social positions, affiliations, roles, and other social categories (Ochs, 1993). Applied linguists have adopted a variety of frameworks to describe how people accomplish these performances and negotiations, including Goffman's (1981) notion of 'footing', Brown and Levinson's (1987) model of politeness, and Sacks' (1995) description of how people use 'membership categorization devices' to orient towards particular 'selves' as relevant to what is going on. What all of these approaches have in common is a commitment to identifying how broader social roles and identities are constructed in the concrete features of discourse.

Positioning

As I said at the start of this chapter, I will be using the term 'positioning' to talk about how people strategically claim and impute social identities in interaction through the appropriation and adaptation of discursive resources from their socio-cultural environments. I am borrowing the term from Rom Harré and his colleagues (Davies and Harré, 1990; Harré and Moghaddam, 2003; Van Langenhove and Harré, 1999) who define it as:

> the discursive process whereby selves are located in conversations as observably and subjectively coherent participants in jointly produced storylines. By giving people parts in a story, whether it be explicit or implicit, a speaker makes available a subject position which the other speaker in the normal course of events would take up.
>
> *(Davies and Harré, 1990, para. 18)*

'Storylines' can be looked at in two ways. On the one hand they can be seen on the local level of the interaction itself, made up of the sequential chains of actions that form the immediate conversational performance. On the other hand they can be seen as made up of already existing expectations about social identities and the social practices associated with them which are part of 'the repertoire of competent members' of a society (Van Langenhove and Harré, 1999, p. 18), what Gee (1996) refers to as 'meta-narratives' and Mishler (1995, 1999) calls 'master narratives'. What is useful about the heuristic offered by Harré and his colleagues is that it gives us a way to see social identities *both* as locally produced and as reflective of broader social structures. It also reminds us that, just as actions occur on multiple simultaneous timescales, so do 'storylines' and the 'selves' that they give rise to. As

Lemke (2000, p. 285) puts it: 'There are longer-term Selves already engaged in on-going longer-term projects and activities, and the shorter-term Selves of current activities, some of which contribute to longer-term projects and some of which may not.'

Finally, the notion of storylines also serves to highlight the underlying *moral* dimension of identity management in interaction. For Harré and his colleagues, when people claim and impute identities, they are always positioning themselves and others not just in relation to each other, but in relation to various 'moral orders' that function on both the local level of the interaction and the broader level of the society or culture. Heritage and Lindstrom (1998) capture this moral dimension of positioning particularly vividly in their analysis of interactions between British health visitors and new mothers. In one encounter they examine, the health visitor asks the following question to an unmarried mother who is living with her boyfriend in her mother's house:

> Uh:m (0.8).hh now first the particulars they want to know th' baby's father's a:ge.
> *(Heritage and Lindstrom, 1998, p. 398)*

As Heritage and Lindstrom point out, through this seemingly simple request for information the health worker positions the mother and herself within a particular moral order. By choosing to refer to the woman's boyfriend as 'th' baby's father', she avoids using the word 'husband', which would be factually incorrect, or the word 'boyfriend', which might highlight the 'illegitimate' status of the child. This compromise term helps the health worker to distance herself from any apparent moral judgment of the woman. At the same time, by positioning herself as asking the question for someone else ('they want to know'), she orients towards the question as intrusive and distances herself from the authorities who have forced her to ask it. Although Heritage and Lindstrom do not explicitly refer to 'storylines', none of the interactional work they describe could be accomplished without participants' sharing a set of 'stories' about things like pregnancy, 'illegitimacy', and bureaucracy.

Another illustration of the moral dimension of positioning can be seen in Fahy and Smith's (1999) description of a conflict between a midwife and obstetrician over the rights and obligations of a teenage woman giving birth, in which the woman is positioned by the doctor as a 'bad mother' when she requests an epidural. When the midwife attempts to intervene, the doctor positions her as unduly (and unprofessionally) influencing the woman's decision. What Fahy and Smith's analysis shows is not just the way people use positioning to assert power over others, but also how particular positions amplify and constrain access by participants to certain discursive resources, thus reproducing and enforcing the 'storylines' from which these positions come.

Positioning and power

Not surprisingly, most treatments of positioning in doctor–patient interactions have been preoccupied with the asymmetrical power relations between participants.

While most approaches to clinical asymmetry from critical sociology and cultural studies (see for example Armstrong, 1982) have viewed it as a reflection of larger social structures and discursive mechanisms – most famously Foucault's (1976) notion of the 'medical gaze' – applied linguistic approaches to power, influenced mostly by conversation analysts, have focused more on how power is *interactionally achieved* through talk. From this perspective the asymmetry in medical encounters is not purely a product of the power that doctors 'bring along' to these interactions. It is also something that is 'brought about' through strategies of questioning, turn-taking, interruption and the like. As West (1984, pp. 95–96) puts it, power and control in medical encounters are best viewed as 'micro-political achievements, produced in and through actual turns at talk.' Institutional structures and other external sources of authority are, of course, not irrelevant. Rather they are viewed both as resources that participants draw upon to negotiate power relations (Maynard, 1991) and as the *consequence* of countless situated social interactions through which they are 'talked into being' (Heritage, 1984, p. 290).

Most studies from this perspective have reinforced the general claim of medical sociology that physicians tend to be highly authoritarian, promulgating their own biomedical models of disease and often undermining patients' experiences and understandings (Maynard, 1991; Mishler, 1984). 'The prototypical example,' as Maynard (1991, p. 450) puts it,

> is of a patient who arrives at a doctor's office and presents a complaint. The doctor, largely by way of questioning strategies that require delimited responses, works the complaint into biomedical categories that lack sensitivity to the patient's psychosocial concerns, life world, and folk understandings.

One of the main ways physicians are able to exercise power is through the discourse positions that they take up (see for example Hodge and Kress, 1988; Scollon, 1998; Zimmerman, 1998). Participants who take up the role of issuing the first part in adjacency sequences in conversations (i.e. asking questions, giving orders, offering advice, etc.), for example, automatically have control over what can coherently be said by the other participant (questions demand answers, orders demand compliance). Physicians' privileged access to this discourse position is in a large part what allows them to assume control over the interaction (Heritage and Greatbatch, 1991). This is the main point made by Byrne and Long (1976) in one of the earliest and most influential interactional studies of medical consultations, in which they found that in three-quarters of the over 2,000 medical interviews they recorded, doctors performed all of the initiating moves and patients all of the responding moves. Subsequent studies have confirmed that moves like questions, orders, and proposals are mostly taken by physicians and seem to be 'dispreferred' when taken by patients (see for example Frankel, 1990; Todd, 1984; West, 1984).

Among the most frequently studied of these initiating moves have been questions. Studies have found that in medical consultations physicians overwhelmingly ask more questions than patients, and that even when patients do ask questions, they are often accompanied by hesitations and other perturbations, and physicians often interrupt them or fail to answer them (Frankel, 1990; West, 1984). Interactional control is maintained by doctors not just through the act of asking questions, but also through the *kinds* of questions they ask, which often restrict the kinds of answers patients can give to short responses (Frankel, 1984a, 1990; Mishler, 1984). Finally, it has been pointed out that physicians also control topics in consultations through how they respond to patients' answers, using 'third turns' in an extremely restrictive way that avoids displaying alignment with the patient or revealing the physician's thought processes. Not surprisingly, physicians' use of 'third turns' to deliver acknowledgments rather than assessments or interpretations can cause anxiety for patients who listen to such turns carefully to figure out what the doctor is making of what they are saying (ten Have, 1991).

Another interactional feature that has played a prominent role in studies of doctor–patient asymmetry is interruptions. An early study by Beckman and Frankel (1984) revealed that doctors interrupted patients on an average of 18 seconds after they started talking, and that once interrupted, patients rarely regained the floor until doctors had issued a further initiating move. In a follow-up study, Beckman, Frankel, and Darnley (1985) found that there was a relationship between interrupted visits and hidden problems expressed by patients at the ends of visits, leading them to express concern that physician interruption had the potential effect of inhibiting patients from supplying information that might be critical for decision-making (see also Henzl, 1989; Roter and Hall, 1992).

An example of how doctors use interruptions to control medical encounters can be seen in the transcript below of a British patient in Hong Kong consulting a bilingual Chinese doctor about a stomach complaint.

01	D:	How can I help you please^
02	P:	umm.I think I have food poisoning =
03	D:	= yeah.what symptoms do you have
04	P:	diarrhea.[uhhh
05	D:	[When did it start^
06	P:	yesterday after[noon
07	D:	(typing) [Any idea how many times.
08		yesterday?
09	P:	Umm.around twenty =
10	D:	= twenty.okay^ (typing)
11	P:	I think [it's^
12	D:	[twenty times
13	P:	at least =
14	D:	= and what about today^
15	P:	today maybe six times =
16	D:	= six times (typing).and is the stool watery [or soft^
17	P:	[it's
18		totally water

19	D:	(typing) any blood^
20	P:	well there's not blood in the [stool I think but
21	D	[in the tissue
22	P:	there's blood [on the eh.eh
23	D:	[blood in the tissue =
24	P:	= it's [umm
25	D:	[sore. so blood in tissue.(typing)
26	P:	It's sore because I'm going to the toilet so [much
27	D:	[there's
28		blood (typing)
29	P:	(.3) yeah
30	D:	in tissue, okay yeah^

In this short excerpt the physician interrupts the patient at least six times, trying to quickly move him through the history-taking part of the consultation as he types the patient's responses into an electronic medical record. At times, in fact, it seems as if the doctor's impatience leads him to force the patient to settle on answers that the patient regards as not entirely satisfactory, as when the doctor insists on recording that there have been twenty incidents of diarrhea when the patient seems anxious to qualify this answer ('around twenty … ', 'I think it's … ', 'at least'). The doctor seems much more satisfied with categorical answers (such as 'totally water') which do not require any further negotiation. There may of course be good reasons for this. For example, there may be time constraints on the doctor regarding how long he can spend with each patient, or institutional constraints as to how answers must be recorded on medical records, and whether or not the patient suffered twenty or twenty-five bouts of diarrhea may indeed be inconsequential. At the same time, this example suggests that one consequence of physician interruption might be to push patients into giving more categorical descriptions of their symptoms and avoiding details or expressions of uncertainty, which in some cases might be relevant to the diagnosis.

Despite the picture of physician 'authoritarianism' suggested by the studies described above, others have pointed out that doctors do not act alone in maintaining asymmetry. Both Heath (1992) and ten Have (1995), for example, have shown how patients sustain their passivity even in stages of the consultation in which physicians actively seek their participation, such as the making of treatment decisions, with some patients refusing outright to contribute. Others have cautioned that studies that use surface features of interactions like questions and interruptions as the only measure of interactional control can end up oversimplifying the issue of power and missing the sometimes subtle ways patients advance their own agendas. As West (1984) herself has pointed out, although patients rarely formulate utterances that take the grammatical form of questions, they do make use of a variety of other ways to show doubt or request further information from doctors such as repetitions, qualification, and paralinguistic or non-verbal cues. Similarly, ten Have (1991) has pointed out how patients sometimes use 'subtle and covert devices' to regain control of topics and 'hold off the doctor's questioning interventions' (p. 142). Finally, Lambert and his colleagues (1997) suggest that as much as physicians are strategic in their use of questions to control the interaction, patients are also strategic in their avoidance of issuing direct questions as a way of positioning themselves as cooperative.

As for interruptions, many of the early studies dealing with this issue failed to take into account the multiple functions interruptions have in conversation. While sometimes we interrupt in order to take the floor from others, at other times interruptions function to express support and encourage the other speaker to continue or elaborate. Studies that have taken this complexity into account, such as that by Aronsson and Sätterlund-Larsson (1987), have found that physician interruptions sometimes function as expressions of eagerness, support, and cooperation, weakening rather than strengthening the asymmetry of the interaction. In a more recent study, Černý (2010, p. 17) found not only that both patients and doctors engaged in an almost equal amount of interrupting, but also that cooperative 'symmetry-oriented' interruptions by both parties outnumbered competitive 'asymmetry-oriented' interruptions.

Finally, not all studies of doctor–patient interactions have revealed the kind of inequality found in the studies cited above. Perhaps the most famous challenge to assumptions of asymmetry in medical encounters comes from Ainsworth-Vaughn (1998), who shows in her analysis of interactions in private medical clinics in the United States that patients often take an active role in co-constructing both their diagnosis and their treatment choices, take the initiative to frame interactions to accommodate their own storytelling, and sometimes openly challenge the assertions and decisions of their physicians. These observations are confirmed by quantitative data, which shows that 40 percent of the questions asked in the encounters studied were asked by patients, a figure that rises to 50 percent in cases in which the doctor was a woman.

At the heart of this debate over whether and how much doctors exert power over patients are two fundamental assumptions about power that limit analysts' capacity to address the complexity of doctor–patient interactions. The first is the assumption that interactional power and 'actual' power are the same thing. This assumption ignores the numerous passive ways patients have of exercising power by, for example, withholding information from the doctor or selectively following his or her instructions. Gabe and Calnan (1989) suggest that behind this apparent asymmetry is often what they call a 'deferential dialectic' in which patients are deferential to doctors because of self-imposed constraints (see also Bell and Newby, 1976), yet maintain an active role in the relationship, evaluating medical practice from their own point of view. The second assumption is that asymmetry is always undesirable. This assumption ignores the fact that in many medical encounters doctors need to exert interactional control in order to be able to effectively look after the well-being of the patient or efficiently work within institutional constraints. It also ignores the fact that many patients themselves feel comfortable with this asymmetry (Silverman, 1987) and may even regard it as 'an implicit part of their treatment' (Gwyn, 2002, p. 74).

The biggest problem with this preoccupation with power and asymmetry in clinical interactions, however, is that power itself is usually not adequately defined beyond surface interactional features. Whereas sociologists taking a macro perspective on power tend to locate it in social structures or in systems of knowledge and ignore how asymmetry is actively achieved by parties in interaction, those who define power chiefly in terms of interactional features such as who asks more questions sometimes ignore the ways power is related to broader social structures and to broader sociocultural notions of the self (Lynch and Bogen, 1994). A focus on 'positioning' rather than 'power' gives us a way to link interactional asymmetry with larger institutional and cultural agendas and to understand how, as (Van Langenhove and Harré, 1999, p. 183, emphasis mine) put it, it is 'the negotiation and adoption of the particular *storylines* that explain and legitimize ... power inequalities'.

'Storylines' of expertise

In some ways, much more enlightening than studies focusing on interactional power have been those which focus on *expertise*, which, after all, is the central warrant for doctors questioning, interrupting and imposing their views on patients. As opposed to studies that focus solely on power, attention to claims and imputations of expertise gives analysts a way to observe how the negotiation of power on the local level is tied to the way participants position themselves in relation to various discourses or 'storylines' of expertise and the communities and institutions that promote these storylines.

Unlike power, which tends to be seen as a kind of finite 'commodity' that participants in interaction compete over, the notion of expertise is more complex. Both healthcare workers and patients bring along to interactions different kinds of expertise and they use claims to expertise (as well as claims to a *lack* of expertise) in various strategic ways. Claims to expertise can be based on access to information, on credentials of various kinds, on membership in particular professions or groups, on affiliation with particular institutions, or on the ability to marshal or interpret certain evidence. While doctors bring to interactions the weight of their cultural authority and credentials, as well as access to specialist information and specific information about patients (such as test results) that patients often do not have access to or the ability to interpret, patients also bring along to interactions their own claims to expertise based on their own experiences and on information they have gleaned from media and conversations with friends, family members, and other experts. With increased access to expert medical knowledge on the internet, some patients come to consultations armed with even more information about a particular condition or drug than their doctors have. This is especially true for patients who have been living with (and learning about) a particular chronic condition for a long period of time, what Sarangi (2010a, p. 304) calls 'professional clients'. The 'progressively less asymmetrical distribution of available knowledge in doctor–patient encounters', Sarangi and Clarke (2002, p. 140) point out, further calls into question Mishler's (1984) dichotomy between the 'voice of medicine' and the 'voice of the lifeworld' (see also Atkinson, 1995; Silverman, 1987).

Most of all, patients are experts on their own lives. They have access to information about their own behavior, living conditions, and symptoms which healthcare workers may need to make an accurate diagnosis or recommend appropriate treatment. While doctors have privileged access to information from things like CT scans and blood tests, patients have privileged access to internal sensations such as pain, dizziness, and nausea, and to signs and symptoms that are no longer present. Moreover, numerous studies (see for example Cole-Kelly, 1992; Jones, et al., 2000) have shown that patients are not only aware of the power associated with this form of expertise but also use it strategically, disclosing different types and different amounts of information to different kinds of healthcare workers.

While doctors and patients 'bring along' different forms of expertise to their encounters, expertise is also something that is 'brought about', that is, claimed, imputed, ratified, and challenged in interaction. In a sense, being an expert requires more than just having a diploma on one's office wall. It requires that one is able to competently perform the role of expert through, for example, being able to produce various kinds of factual or evidential accounts of phenomena, to manage assessments of probability, to control conversational topics, to manage politeness strategies and the alignment of frames, and to make use of indirectness, mitigation, hedging, and other rhetorical devices (Candlin and Candlin, 2002). It also involves knowing when it is appropriate to assume different discourse positions in interaction, when one should, for example, ask, instruct, advise, prohibit, or persuade. At the same time, claiming expertise puts one in the special position of having to *account* for one's decisions and actions in ways that non-experts do not. Heritage (2005) observes, for example, that the degree to which doctors are willing to claim expertise depends a great deal on how much they need to or are able to account for how they have arrived at their decisions. Similarly, Peräkylä (1998) has observed that even when patients are not equipped to understand or evaluate the explanations given by doctors, doctors are still socially obligated to offer such explanations (see also Peräkylä, 2002).

Of course, the discursive resources available in interaction for doctors and patients to claim expertise are unequally distributed, so that when patients do things like offering a self-diagnosis, they usually must do so within the framework or 'storyline' defined by the doctor (Peräkylä, 2002). At the same time, the doctor's position as an expert cannot be established alone: it requires the ratification of the patient (a ratification which, with the increased circulation of medical knowledge on the internet and growing suspicions about the medical profession in some circles, is not always a given). Whether we are speaking of the expertise of the doctor or the expertise of the patient, 'the discursive expression of expertise is to different extents a co-participative endeavor of all involved' (Candlin and Candlin, 2002, p. 116).

A good example of how doctors and patients claim different kinds of expertise and how this affects the way they interpret evidence can be seen in Moore, Plum and Candlin's (2001) study of how HIV positive patients and their doctors talk about 'viral load' (the amount of HIV present in a blood sample based on laboratory tests). 'Viral load', they argue, means something different in the context of the 'discourse of health measurement', in which it is seen as an objective property of the HIV-infected body, the 'discourse of healthcare', in which it is seen primarily as an indicator of treatment effectiveness and/or of patient (non)-compliance, and the 'discourse of health experience', in which it is seen as a matter of the subjective experiences of the patient. All three of these different discourses make available different positions of expertise and, as Moore and her colleagues point out, this can sometimes result in conflicting interpretations and misaligned views between doctors and patients. Such misalignments, they claim, are not just a matter of conflicting opinions, but a matter of conflicting 'storylines' in which 'viral load' plays a part. At the same time, it would be a mistake to assume that doctors always take up positions of expertise within the discourses of health measurement or healthcare and that patients always stake their claims to expertise on subjective experiences. In fact, one of the most interesting things about the study by Moore and her colleagues is that it demonstrates how *all three* of these storylines are available to both doctors and patients, and how, at different points in the interaction, different parties might take up positions in different discourses, patients sometimes claiming expertise in the medical model by 'talking the numbers' with their doctors, and doctors demonstrating empathy by invoking the storyline of the patient's subjective experience.

The main point here is that positions of expertise that are taken up in medical interactions by doctors and patients are not just a matter of power asymmetry in the conventional sense. Indeed, in the interactions that Moore and her colleagues examined, the position of expertise claimed by the patient based on his lived experiences often trumped the more 'academic' expertise of the doctor. What is important in such negotiations is not the interactional power of either the doctor or the patient, but rather the dominance of particular storylines of expertise. In almost all of the encounters analyzed by Moore and her colleagues, one of these storylines of expertise emerged as dominant. What is at stake, then, in negotiations of expertise between doctors and patients is not just 'who's right and who's wrong', but how different storylines of expertise 'connect with each other: how they correspond, how they counter each other, how they cut across each other, and when necessary, which gives way' (Moore et al., 2001, p. 445).

'Trading places'

One place where the fluid and strategic nature of positioning in health related encounters is particularly evident is moments when participants effectively invite their interlocutors to 'trade' positions with them, when patients ask doctors to put themselves in the position of patients and doctors ask patients to put themselves in the position of doctors.

One example of patients asking doctors or other healthcare professionals to trade places with them is when they ask what has come to be referred to as 'the famous-infamous question': some variant of 'What would you do if you were me?' In such cases, healthcare workers are often put into the difficult position of maintaining their position of expertise while avoiding compromising the decision-making position of the patient or client. Sarangi and Clarke (2002, p. 160; see also Sarangi, 2000) give a good example of how a genetic counselor strategically avoids taking up this position when it is offered by a client in the excerpt below.

[D = Doctor; H = Husband; W = Wife]

01	H:	so it it eh to cut a long story short, if eh your wife was in this
02		position God forbid (.5) eh and you wanted another child would
03		you say (.) the chances are so minute (.5) we can go ahead with
04		one? (.5)
05	H:	it was your-
06	D:	[you're asking-(.) you're asking (.) two separate questions
07	H:	[if you were me or-
08	D:	yeah
09	H:	= well yeah
10	D:	but you're you *are* asking two separate questions
11	H:	mmh
12	D:	you see there's the (.) the (.) the you know what you're saying
13		one is (.) eh (.) is there a chance of eh (.) say of a child having a
14		tendency to get meningiomas?
15	H:	[^^^^^] (.) well I know I know it's like it would be the
16		same chances as some [^^^^^]
17	D:	yes that's very very unlikely
18	H:	[unlikely
19	D:	[so there's *that* question. and then there is the question of
20	H:	mhm
21	D:	of would the pregnancy *cause* another tumor (1.0)
22	D	and (.) I think the answer [to that
23	H:	[that's unclear
24	D:	= well I think (.) the pregnancy itself wouldn't cause another
25		tumor. (.) if there is a small recurrence eh that (.) was not
26		identified on the scan (.) then I suppose a pregnancy could
27		perhaps influence that rate of growth but (.) it's not going to
28		make the difference between (.) the tumor coming back or not
29		coming back. (.5) it (.5) could make a (.) a difference to when it
30		shows itself.

As Sarangi and Clarke point out, the dilemma the counselor finds himself in here is not so much having to take up the position of a husband with a wife with a tumor (God forbid!), but with having to take up the position of personal advisor rather than information-provider and decision-facilitator. The way he wriggles out of this position is by asserting his expertise in information-giving, first by 'analyzing' and reframing the husband's question ('you're asking two separate questions'), and then answering in an objective way which allows him to assert his medical expertise as opposed to his expertise as a hypothetical husband.

An important point that Sarangi and Clark make in their analysis of such reversals is that, despite the fact that they often make professionals uncomfortable, they do serve important strategic functions for patients and clients, often in cases where patients wish to reduce their uncertainty through soliciting expert advice. In other words, what is often behind such invitations to 'put yourself in my place' is a desire for the expert to do just the opposite: to offer explicit advice from their position of professional expertise.

Of course not all healthcare professionals avoid taking up the position of the patient when invited to do so. Willingness to take up this position, however, seems to be related to how secure they feel in their own position of professional expertise. Barton (2007, p. 32) gives an example from an interaction in which a doctor is involved in recruiting a patient for a clinical trial for a cancer drug:

01	Mrs. G:	Let me ask you what I consider an important question.
02		Are you married?
03	Dr. T:	Yeah.
04	Mrs. G:	If it were your wife would you have her do this, if she
05		had my cancer?
06	Dr. T:	I'd have her try.
07	Mrs. G:	What if it was your mother, because I don't know the
08		relationship you have with your wife ((*laughter*)).
09	Dr. T:	I would encourage her to at least try. I would be
10		disappointed if I honestly didn't get the [drug], but that's
11		the other standard. You don't get anything anyways, so
12		there's no losing to me.

Here the patient attempts to reduce her uncertainty about participating in the trial by positioning herself in a hypothetical intimate relationship with the doctor, first as his wife and then as his mother, to check if he would still recommend participating. Unlike the genetic counselor above, the doctor in this situation does not hesitate to take up the position offered and use it to model the kind of decision-making process he wishes her to perform. One reason for this may be that the decision seems less ambiguous to the doctor – perhaps by participating in the trial the patient truly has everything to gain and nothing to lose. A more cynical interpretation would consider the possible benefits the doctor might accrue from the pharmaceutical company for signing up more patients for the trial, and cynical as it is, this perspective points to a possible reason for such repositionings that is often ignored in the literature: the way such questions may serve as a patient's way of testing the underlying motivation of the doctor for making certain recommendations.

Just as patients sometimes invite doctors to take on the role of patients (or patients' relatives), doctors sometimes invite patients to take on the role of doctors. The most famous treatment of this phenomenon is Maynard's (1991) description of the use of the 'perspective display series' in clinical encounters. The 'perspective display series' is a common move in ordinary conversation in which a speaker invites his or her interlocutor to give an opinion or assessment before delivering his or her own opinion or assessment. Normally such a move allows the speaker to gauge how the other will respond to his or her view and to tailor their speech in a way that creates the impression of a mutuality of perspective between the two parties. According to Maynard, this strategy is quite common in clinical interactions, often serving as a way of preparing for bad news or laying the groundwork for acceptance of a diagnosis or compliance with a treatment. In his seminal paper on this phenomenon, Maynard analyzes the interaction between healthcare workers and parents at a pediatric clinic specializing in developmental disorders, an example of which is given below.

01	Dr. E:	What do you see? as as- his difficulty.
02	Mrs. C:	Mainly his uhm- the fact that he doesn't understand
03		everything and also the fact that his speech is very hard
04		to understand what he's saying, lots of time
05	Dr. E:	Right
06	Dr. E:	Do you have any ideas WHY it is? are you- do you?
07	Mrs. C:	No
08	Dr. E:	Okay I you know I think we BASICALLY in some ways
09		agree with with you, insofar as we think that D's MAIN
10		problem, you know DOES involve you know LANGuage,
11	Mrs. C:	Mm hmm
12	Dr. E:	you know both you know his- being able to
13		underSTAND, and know what is said to him, and also
14		certainly also to be able to express, you know his uh
15		thoughts (1.0)
16	Dr. E:	Um, in general his development …

(Maynard, 1991, p. 468)

In this excerpt the doctor invites the child's mother to offer her own assessment of her child's behavior and her own opinion about its cause before delivering his diagnosis, and when the diagnosis is finally given, it is linked to the parent's diagnosis ('you know I think we BASICALLY in some ways agree with with you … '). In this way, the doctor makes the diagnosis seem like a shared enterprise between the doctor and the parent and prepares the mother to accept aspects of the doctor's assessment that might be different from her own. There are, of course, lots of good medical reasons for using such a strategy, particularly in questions involving childhood developmental issues in which behavior observed at home might be highly relevant to the diagnosis. At the same time, there are also good *discursive* reasons for using this strategy since, by co-implicating the parent in the assessment, the doctor promotes the appearance of agreement between the two parties and preempts possible challenges.

In other words, just as patients' invitations to doctors to take the position of patients or patients' loved ones are often designed to get doctors to act more like doctors (to be more forthcoming with their expert advice), doctors' invitations to patients or patients' surrogates to take the position of doctors are often actually designed to get them to act more like patients (and accept what the doctor is going to tell them).

Another example can be seen in the following transcript from Sarangi's (2010b) study of the strategies doctors use to avoid prescribing antibiotics.

01	GP:	Hello, there
02	P:	Hi
03	GP:	Hi, what can we do for Lincoln?
04	P:	It's both of them really, she's had what I thought was a cold
05		since Friday, but I just kept putting it off, putting it off, but the
06		cough just seems to be getting worse, and he's got it as well, so
07		I'm not sure if they've got some sort of infection
08	GP:	Right, who shall we look at first? Little one, so he's got a cough?
09		Anything else you've noticed wrong with him?
10	P:	No, he hasn't been too bad, but she hasn't been eating though
11	GP:	Snuffy nose, temperature, and that stuff?
12	P:	Yes they've had high temperatures, I mean, they're obviously
13		together, so
14	GP:	All right, anybody else had it?
15	P:	No
16	GP:	Just the kids
17	P:	Yeah, feverish, cold
18	GP:	Right, and what do you think is going on, you mentioned a cold?
19		What is it that worries you, something more … ?
20	P:	Well, they've been up until (unclear), they've been really
21		uncomfortable with the coughing, so I started to think, you
22		know whether they had a throat infection
23	GP:	Right, okay, and what did you think I might do with them today,
24		did you have any ideas about how we would deal with that?
25	P:	No … (unclear) … antibiotics

(Sarangi, 2010b, p. 90)

In this excerpt, the main reason for the doctor eliciting the parent's medical opinion seems to be to prepare the ground for the non-prescription of antibiotics. The way he does this is both by eliciting a direct request for antibiotics, which he can then address directly, and by also eliciting the parent's opinion that the symptoms are due to a 'cold' (a condition not treatable with antibiotics). One important point that we can take from these two examples, then, is that when doctors do elicit assessments from patients, they are often very selective about what aspects of those assessments they take up in delivering their own opinions, often choosing to emphasize those aspects of the patient's opinion that will support their own judgments ('you mentioned a cold').

There are other situations in which patients engage in 'doctor' talk or when doctors align themselves with patients that are not invited. Patients, for example, might proactively engage in biomedical discourse in order to assert their expertise or challenge the doctor's authority, or doctors might align themselves with patients in opposition to medical orthodoxy. In contrast to the example above, where the doctor solicits the patient's opinion in order to prepare the ground for the non-prescription of antibiotics, in the following example, a continuation of the interaction between the expatriate patient and local doctor in Hong Kong discussed earlier, the doctor invites the patient to join him in an almost conspiratorial relationship against 'by the book' medicine in favor of the prescription of antibiotics.

81	D:	(typing) now.ah.the treatment have two
82		choices (.5) now according to the book we need to
83		get some stool to test before we start antibiotic
84		okay^ (.5) but because your diarrhea is very
85		significant (.5) now: some people prefer to start
86		antibiotic rather than waiting for the stool sample.
87		forget about the stool.because it's difficult to
88		surren.to surrender the stool anyway okay^ (.8)
89		so.what is your choice^.you want to do the proper
90		way^ or the shortcut way.of course it's not
91		textbook =
92	P:	= yeah I think perhaps the shortcut [is uh
93	D:	I[yes sure
94		I'd do the same myself but I need to explain
95		to you what are the pros and cons okay^

Although the doctor here presents to the patient the 'proper', 'textbook' alternative of analyzing a stool sample before prescribing antibiotics, it is by his very use of words like 'proper' and 'textbook' that he signals to the patient his dispreference for this choice and his endorsement of the 'shortcut', an endorsement which he makes explicit when he puts himself in the position of the patient ('I'd do the same myself').

What I have been trying to demonstrate with these examples is that the issues of power and asymmetry in medical encounters are not as simple as they may at first seem. In such encounters, multiple positions of power and expertise are available to both doctors and patients, and they assume, surrender, defend and impute these positions strategically in order to reach particular goals. In most cases, displaying 'expertise' is more than just being able to show one's command of a particular body of knowledge; indeed, as Sarangi and Clarke (2002) note, in some situations claiming expertise has to do more with how one displays uncertainty than knowledge. Further, as laypeople have more access to medical knowledge, traditional positions of expertise become more complex and tenuous. Sarangi and Clarke (2002) see clinical encounters as a matter of professionals and laypeople positioning themselves within and across various 'zones of expertise' (Sarangi and Clarke, 2002) whose borders are constantly shifting as professions become more and more narrowly specialized and patients become more and more 'professional'.

Framing and positioning in discussions about risk

As can be seen from the discussion above, talking about risk in medical encounters often takes place in the context of multiple, sometimes overlapping activities such as giving information, giving advice, instructing, and persuading, and also involves healthcare workers and patients taking on multiple identities as they position themselves within different 'zones of expertise'.

In the last chapter I discussed how risk is discursively constructed through various processes of entextualization through which 'risky practices' and 'risky people' are 'technologized'. In face-to-face interactions risk is similarly subject to the effects of the different discursive strategies people use to represent it, to manage their relationships, and to organize their interactions.

The main problem with talking about risk in practically any context is that it is a fundamentally face-threatening act (Myers, 2003). In medical encounters it almost always involves positioning the patient as personally 'at risk', and also often involves calling into question his or her personal behavior, lifestyle, or integrity (Linell et al., 2002). While talk about risk is risky for patients, it is also risky for healthcare professionals, who not only face the discomfort of having to deliver 'bad news', but also put themselves in the position of potentially having to defend their risk assessments.

The following excerpt from a study by Sarangi on the interaction between genetic counselors and their clients illustrates the awkwardness that often accompanies discussions of risk as well as some of the strategies people use to deal with it.

```
01   G2:   now I did this for your (.) for your family and we do it using a
02         computer (.5) but it's essentially just sort of a complicated
03         calculation
04   AF:   yes
05   G2:   and your own risk is higher than that of the general population =
06   AF:   I thought it would be ((tense laugh)) I'm not surprised
07   G2:   thought yeah yeah it's it's your risk is about thirty percent
08         basically
09         I [think] so you're^^^^^^^a thirty [percent
10   AF:   [so that's high high is it? Or:
11   G2:   it's (.5) it is
12   AF:   yeah
13   G2:   significantly high I mean anything that we're-I mean w-
14   AF:   erm
15   G2    has to be taken with a pinch of salt because it is
16   AF:   yeah:ah
```

17	G2:	just based on a sort of mathematical calculations so it's not
18		a (.5) a
19	AF:	yeah:ah
20	G2:	figure [that is set
21	AF:	[no: no:
22	G2:	in stone or anything [like that that-
23	AF:	[erm
24	G2:	so it would mean that sort of three times out of ten you would
25		Have a chance of (.) breast cancer (.) but then again seven
26		times out of ten you won't [develop breast cancer
27	AF:	[*yes:* (.5)
28	G2:	so you-(.5) so your chance is about three times as high as
29		the general population
30	AF:	oh that's nice ((laughing)) [hhh hhhhh hhhhh hah hah
31	G2:	[^^^ ^ na:
32	G2:	but it (.) it sounds like that's not a lot (.5) not a big (.5)
33	G2:	of a [of a yeah yeah
34	AF:	[oh it's no *shock* no no
35	G2:	(you thought that it'd go up higher) (.5) you *would* be (1.0)
36		we *would* think about seriously think about looking for a gene
37		in your family [(^^ ^^)
38	AF:	[mhm

(Sarangi, 2010a, p. 185)

One of the most striking things about this excerpt is the way the genetic counselor continually modulates and qualifies her assessment of the client's risk. As Sarangi puts it, the escalation and de-escalation of the seriousness of the risk follows a kind of rhythmic, 'dance-like' pattern, where every escalation is followed in the next turn by a de-escalation. This comparison to a dance is particularly apt when we consider that these alternations of escalation and de-escalation are apparently motivated by the patient's responses, which follow a similar pattern of concern ('so that's *high high* is it?') and (albeit rather forced) dismissiveness ('it's no *shock* no no'). In other words, the client's risk of breast cancer in this excerpt is co-constructed by the counselor and the client through various small acts of framing and reframing: the doctor, for example, reframing the client's risk from a three out of ten chance of developing breast cancer to a seven out of ten chance of *not* developing it, and the client, for example, attempting to mitigate the effects of the bad news on both herself and the counselor by framing it as 'old news'. There are also various small acts of repositioning, as the counselor alternately asserts the accuracy of her assessment and the uncertainty associated with it through the use of hedges and modal verbs, and the patient alternately presents herself as worried and unsurprised.

One of the most interesting aspects of this excerpt is the way the counselor characterizes the text through which the discussion of risk is mediated. Discussions of risk in clinical encounters are often mediated through texts of the kind discussed in the last chapter. As I noted in that discussion, different kinds of texts impose different affordances and constraints on how risk can be talked about. These affordances and constraints themselves, however, do not wholly determine how such texts can be used in sites of engagement. Also important are the strategic ways participants appropriate and adapt them to meet particular interactional goals. In the example above, the report undergoes a kind of transformation as the counselor appropriates it as a tool for escalating and de-escalating her risk assessment: it begins as something involving a 'computer', and is then revised to something seemingly less 'high tech' ('essentially just sort of a complicated calculation'), later becoming a source of precise statistics ('you're ... a thirty percent'), and still later being again demoted to something whose relevance and veracity are seen as questionable ('it *is* ... just based on a sort of mathematical calculations so it's not a ... figure that is set in stone or anything like that').

Adelswärd and Sachs (1998) observe similar kinds of strategies in their study of how doctors and patients recontextualize epidemiological risk calculations in clinical encounters. Often, they note, physicians frame and reframe statistical information with reference to 'ideals', 'means', and 'limits', while patients similarly attempt to use such figures to determine how 'normal' they are. Such strategies help participants avoid assessments like 'high' or 'low' or 'good' or 'bad'.

How participants in medical encounters communicate about risk depends a great deal on how they frame 'risk talk' as an activity and what role it takes in the wider activity of the interaction. Often talk about risk is framed as something else altogether, sometimes in an attempt to avoid alarming the patient or delivering a risk assessment prematurely. In the following excerpt from a study by Adolphs and her colleagues (2007), the nurse, faced with the need to ask the patient about meningitis symptoms, which might lead to a potentially serious diagnosis, attempts to mitigate the threat of the risk talk by reframing the activity as an administrative rather than a medical task: it is the requirements of the form that are responsible for the imputation of the risk, not the judgment of the nurse.

01	NHS Nurse:	cos we have to *kind of* un = we = we always
02		do *like* the worst case scenario and work downwards
03	Patient:	all right ((laughs)) okay
04	NHS Nurse:	we always like look at the *meningitis type symptoms*
05		first
06	Patient:	yeah
07	NHS Nurse:	okay and then we work downwards (.) so just bear with
08		me

(Adolphs et al., 2007, p. 67)

What is also at stake when people talk about risk is the different status of the participants in the talk, the degree to which they are positioned as 'at-risk' or 'safe', as 'agents' in causing the situation or as 'innocent victims', as 'empowered' to take action in response to the risk or 'helpless' in the face of it, and as 'entitled' to talk about risk from within different 'zones of expertise'.

One of the consequences of advances in medical technology that allow for earlier and more accurate detection of medical anomalies is that more and more people who before would have been considered 'healthy' are now positioned as patients. Rather than being seen as an abstract calculation of the probability of future events, risk has become something that people 'have'. As Linell and his colleagues (2002, p. 201) put it, 'When risks get talked about in individualized terms, they tend to become concretized, almost reified as if they were something "carried" by the patient in her own body' (see also Adelswärd and Sachs, 1998). It is a short step from seeing risk as a property of an individual to seeing that individual as *embodying* risk ('so you're ... a thirty percent').

An important aspect of risk talk in clinical settings, then, is managing the imputation of 'risky-identities'. As I noted above, professionals and patients use a variety of linguistic resources like hedging, modal verbs and displays of surprise or nonchalance to position themselves in relation to risk assessments. Sometimes these discursive tools can be even subtler and more delicate. In a classic study of the imputation of 'at risk' identities in counseling sessions at an HIV testing center, Silverman and Peräkylä (D. Silverman, 1997; Silverman and Peräkylä, 1990), for example, demonstrate how seemingly insignificant features in conversation such as pauses, hesitations, and false starts can be used to mitigate the possible face threats associated with imputing 'at risk' identities. In the counseling sessions they analyzed, they noticed that nearly all such imputations were marked by verbal perturbations (such as hesitations). The excerpt below shows an example of this:

```
03   C:   (0.4) can I just ask you briefly (0.2) erm: one or two questions
04        before we start hh have you ever had a test before?
05   P:   no
06   C:   no hhh have you ever injected drugs?
07   P:   no
08   C:   (2.0) have you ever had a homosexual relationship?
09   P:   (0.5) no (0.5) and that's not really (0.5) (I mean) (0.2)
10        put me in a high risk group now [has it?
11   C:   [no
```

(Silverman and Peräkylä, 1990, p. 296)

In this excerpt there is a clear contrast between the way the counselor asks the first two questions (lines 4–7), preceding them only with slight in-breaths, and how she asks the third question (line 8), which is preceded by a pause of two full seconds. The client also uses pauses to mark the topic as delicate, and then, in contrast to the previous short answer, produces an elaborated interpretation of the question as a way of further distancing himself from any imputation of risk.

The imputation of 'at risk' identity is not the only face threat in risk-counseling situations. Sometimes the imputation of 'low risk' identity can be equally threatening, especially when it denies a client the psychological stability of a long-held 'at risk' identity (along with the various social practices that support such an identity), or makes it more difficult to access goods and services which an 'at risk' identity makes available. Sarangi (2010b) gives an example of this in his analysis of a genetic counseling session focused on breast cancer risks:

```
01    GC:    women who have the faulty gene, by her age we'd say at least
02           two thirds of them would have had cancer by now
03    CL:    yes
04    GC:    yeah (pause) I'm not sure whether you're going to be pleased
05           about this or not, but I think you're in the group of women that
06           we'd think are low risk ((pause))
07    CL:    oh right
08    GC:    mm (.) and therefore I think you're in the group of women for
09           whom we'd say probably additional screening is not necessary.
10    CL:    ri:ght
                                      *
13    GC:    em (.) I mean having (.) said that, what's going through your
14           mind now (.) is it sort of like – ((pause))
15    CL:    ehm ((pause)) ((exhales, sighs)) *pf:::::::* (.) I-
16           I (don't feel) very comfortable with it, I almost
17           felt like > > uh I wish I hadn't come then < <
18    GC:    mm
19    CL:    because I had my mammogram every year
20    GC:    yeah
21    CL:    but ehn ((pause))
```

(Sarangi, 2010b, p. 409)

Here we can see the same pattern of pauses and perturbations preceding the categorization of the patient into a 'low-risk' group that we saw above with the potential categorization of a client into a 'high-risk' group. We also see the use of hedges and modal verbs ('I think … ', 'we'd say probably') we would normally associate with the softening of 'bad news' rather than the delivery of 'good news'. This last example reminds us that when it comes to discussions of risk we cannot rely on simple assumptions that 'high risk' is 'bad' and 'low risk' is 'good'. In clinical settings, and especially in the kinds of non-clinical encounters I will be discussing in the next chapter, the social values assigned to risk are highly variable and context-dependent: sometimes what professionals consider to be the source of risk may be very different from what their clients do. For the woman in the excerpt above, for example, the risk of losing access to her yearly mammograms and the comfort she derives from them seems actually more serious than the risk of breast cancer itself.

Risk and expertise

One important way participants in clinical settings manage the difficulties associated with risk talk is the way they position themselves as more or less 'entitled' to talk about risk based on various claims and imputations of expertise. As I mentioned above in my discussion of the study by Moore and her colleagues (2001) of HIV positive patients talking to their doctors, patients can sometimes challenge assessments of risk offered by professionals by asserting their own 'expertise' as the ultimate arbiters of 'how they feel':

82	P:	But I feel all right so y'know that's the main thing isn't it?
83	D:	Yes ... that's halfway there.
84	P:	Yeah well this is only part of the picture isn't it?
85	D:	Exactly.
86	P:	If I was feeling lousy I'd be concerned, but since I don't ...

(Moore et al., 2001, p. 433)

How much one is willing and able to talk about risk, then, has a lot to do with the kinds of identities one 'brings along' to medical encounters. For patients this might involve their previous experience with the risk under discussion or their membership in a particular community or 'risk group'. For professionals it has to do with their membership in particular 'professional discourse systems' (see chapter 8). Professionals of different kinds may have different access to information or different perspectives on what constitutes 'high', 'low', or 'normal' risk. Professionals are also members of institutions with their own rules or conventions about who is authorized to communicate about risk (for example, doctors usually command a greater entitlement to make assessments about risk than nurses), and the kinds of resources that can be used to address different kinds of risk.

Positions of expertise and 'authority' to talk about risk are not just 'brought along' to such encounters; they are also actively negotiated by the parties involved, often as a way of accomplishing particular interactional goals. Sarangi and Clark (2002), for example, describe how genetic counselors use 'risk talk' to delineate their 'zones of expertise' in order to avoid taking directive, 'advice-giving' positions and to shield themselves from responsibility for their assessments. In genetic counseling sessions, they note, there is an inherent 'tension between clients seeking an authoritative, definitive risk assessment and the geneticist-expert actively defining the boundaries of his or her (in)expertise through formulation of uncertainty' (p. 139). This tension can be seen in the following excerpt where the counselor attempts to avoid giving a definitive answer to a client's questions about the risk of a tumor reoccurring:

01	D:	yeah. 'cause I don't I don't think there's any reason to think
02		that (.) a pregnancy could (.) eh (.) make the difference between
03		a recurrence or not a recurrence (.5) I think (.) it might not- I
04		suppose it *might* influence the rate of growth of a proper (.) eh
05		tumor (.) so that if there was a small recurrence then it might
06		show itself a little bit sooner. (.) but that's only a a might (.) and
07		eh (.).hhh I think really from the point of view of the tumor you

08		had (.) I think the normal MRI scan you've had since this (.)
09		offers you a lot of reassurance (0.7) eh (.) and (.) I don't I don't
10		think I am really I'm in-(0.7) I am in I'm not in a good position
11		to (.) to *advise* and the I think Mr (name)-(.) the neurosurgeons
12		(.) you know (.) are going to have a much better (.)
13	W:	mmh
14	D:	idea as to how *likely* it is to come back (.) and if Mr. (name) is
15		fairly confident (.) that he managed to remove it all, and if the
16		MRI scan has been normal then hhhh (0.5)
17	W:	I don't know *why* he said that he maybe (.) ehm you know it's
18		all confused

(Sarangi and Clarke, 2002, p. 150)

Here we can see many of the discursive features discussed above – hedges, hesitations, modal verbs – which the counselor uses to communicate his uncertainty to the patient. Along with these, the counselor also explicitly defers to other colleagues with expertise in other areas. In doing this, the counselor manages both to avoid taking a directive stance and to avoid directly contradicting other experts. What is interesting about such expressions of uncertainty is that, rather than compromising the counselor's position of expertise, they seem to reinforce it, giving to his assertions a greater weight of authority.

*

In this chapter I discussed some of the complexities involved in understanding communication between health professionals and their patients in clinical situations. I discussed the different ways doctors and patients negotiate sequential, interactive and temporal frames, and how they position themselves in relation to various 'storylines of expertise'. I then applied these concepts to a discussion of talk about risk in professional encounters. In the next chapter, I will show how many of the same tools that have been developed for the analysis of professional communication can also be brought to bear on the analysis of everyday talk about risk.

5

BEYOND THE CLINIC

The scene is a playground in Hong Kong in the middle of the night. A group of teenagers stagger in the darkness, playing on swings and hanging from monkey bars, their laughing faces flashing in the streetlamps while ominous music plays in the background. Two younger boys approach and gaze at them through the fence. 'Hey,' says one of the teenagers to them. 'Feeling bored?' He holds out his hand to reveal a white tablet resting in his palm. 'Try one. Nothing will happen to you.' Just as one of the younger boys is reaching out to take the tablet, an older boy appears from behind. 'Don't try,' he says. 'It'll ruin your life!' They turn around and begin to walk away as a baritone voiceover intones: 'Be smart! Say no to drugs.'

> 'So fucking lame!' exclaims Natalie, lying on the sofa in front of the TV screen in the youth center.
> 'Do you think that guy looks like Brian?' asks her friend.
> 'No fucking way!'
> 'So you didn't find that one effective?' asks the researcher.
> 'No way,' says Natalie.
> 'It's nothing like that in real life,' offers Ah Sing, a boy sitting in the armchair next to her.
> 'Don't try,' shouts Natalie in a mocking voice. 'Say no to drugs! Nobody talks like that.'
> 'In real life they would have killed that guy,' Ah Sing deadpans.
> 'I still think he looks a little like Brian,' Natalie's friend offers.
>
> *(Jones, 1999)*

*

'I can remember exactly the night we stopped using condoms,' said Jason, 'but I can't really say why. It just sort of happened, like some sort of silent agreement, and we haven't used them since. For me, safe sex was always just something that you just did. Every time you went out to a club, there were condoms everywhere. You didn't question it. And we did use them for the first couple of weeks we were together. But then one night we didn't. At first I was like, "Hmmm, not good." But then the next time, I didn't give it a second thought. We never talked about it. We both have sex with other people, so I guess as long as we use condoms with them, then it's okay.'

*

As I noted in the last chapter, most of the research on situated interactions around health and risk has taken place in doctors' offices, clinics, and hospitals. The anecdotes above, however, dramatically illustrate the fact that many of the most important interactions we have around health and risk take place outside of such settings and involve people who are not health professionals, but rather friends, acquaintances, family members, and sexual partners. These non-professional interactions – what Brown and his colleagues (2006, p. 95) call 'wildtrack' communication – are almost always more influential in determining the concrete actions we take around health and risk than interactions with doctors, partly because what is often happening in them is the actual negotiation of risk behavior in 'real time'. They are the moments when the man with high cholesterol decides whether or not to reach for another helping of ice cream, when the teenager decides whether or not to accept the joint that has been passed to him at a party, and when the couple decides whether or not to use a condom.

As we saw in the last chapter, many discussions of health and risk in clinical settings are presented in the abstract, generalized terms and mathematical probabilities which have become the currency of 'evidence based medicine', terms and probabilities which do not always take into account the individual circumstances of patients as they navigate health and risk 'in the wild'. Outside of the clinic, however, interactions around health and risk are always embedded within a multitude of complex social activities and within a web of complex social relationships, and it is impossible to account for people's health behavior without taking into account these activities and relationships. In the study I conducted on the communication between HIV infected patients and their doctors in Hong Kong, which I referred to in chapter 2 (Jones et al., 2000), for example, one of the main sources of miscommunication between doctors and patients centered on patients' failure to adhere to their medication regimens. Doctors interpreted this failure in medical terms, assuming either that patients did not understand how to take their medicines or that they were experiencing side effects which made taking the medicines more difficult. Their responses to patients' missing doses, therefore, focused on providing them with more information or trying to determine the kinds of side effects they were experiencing.

The patients' explanations of their failure to take their pills the way they were supposed to, on the other hand, often had more to do with the social circumstances in which they found themselves when they had to take the medicine. Since some of their medicines had to be taken either immediately before or immediately after eating, these circumstances often involved mealtimes with friends or family members who were not aware of their condition, and so patients had to find ways to conceal the fact that they were taking medicine or delay the dose until a more convenient moment. Although the dynamics of mealtimes with family and friends might seem only peripherally related to a person's ability to comply with a treatment regimen, many of the Chinese HIV patients we talked to regarded this as a major obstacle.

Here it is important to note that when dealing with risk in situated social interactions, what doctors and other professionals see as 'risky' (missing doses of medicine, engaging in unsafe sex, taking illegal drugs) is not always the same as what participants in these interactions see as 'risky' (letting family members know they are HIV positive, making a spouse or sexual partner angry or suspicious, getting into a fight with a gang of older kids).

What we talk about when we talk about health

Interactions around health and risk outside of the clinic, just as those I discussed in the last chapter that occur within clinics and hospitals, are ultimately about 'what we are doing' and 'who we are being'. When we offer someone drugs, ask them to put on a condom, or engage in any other action with consequences for our health, we are always doing so within the context of some social activity and some set of social relationships. At the same time, such offers, requests, and actions themselves function to *create* social situations and *claim* and *impute* social identities.

Talking about 'mom's cancer'

In a pioneering study of the dynamics of health-related communication within families, Beach (2001, 2009) shows how discussions of a mother's cancer invariably involve family members in interactions in which the topic of 'mom's cancer' becomes a vehicle for talking about many other things. The problems inherent in discussing our own or others' health status in the context of families, Beach argues, have to do not just with the difficulties in translating 'medical issues' into the language of 'everyday life', but also with the fact that, when embedded in 'everyday lives', conversations about 'medical issues' invariably get tied up with a host of 'non-medical' storylines. One of the examples he gives is a phone conversation between the son of a woman who is dying of cancer (S) and his ex-wife (G) in which he updates her on his mother's condition.

```
01   S:    hello Doug here
02   G:    I lov:e yo:u:
03   S:    hi
```

```
04   G:   I wanted to tell you tha:t =
05   S:   = well tha:n[ks
06   G:   [(you're the one)
07        (0.2)
08   S:   hhh thanks hhh
09   G:   you're the () one, I [know that]
10   S:   [.hhh] thanks
11   G:   (loved him)
12   S:   .hhhh hhhh well there's a po:ssibility I might
13        not be coming now
14   G:   why?
15   S:   pt oh-hh.hh [because –] [well =
16   G:   [()] pull t[(hrough)^
17   S:   = not pulling thro:gh but at least s:ta:bilized = an:d
18        of course I can only be gone so: lo:ng = so.hhh if it
19        looks like she's gonna (.) hang in for another (0.2)
20        couple of wee:ks^ then I'll wanna wait a couple of
21        weeks but =
22   G:   = oh my g(h)o[:d ((laughter))
23   S:   [ye:ah ri:ght.hh uhm, hh so that's
24        in fact that's what I thought this pho:ne call was, =
25        I'm – I'm waiting, (.) to hear from, =
26   G:   = () did they call you last ni:ght^
27   S:   yeah
28        (1.2)
29   S:   yeah we – e – u:m – pt a:nd she's gotta.hhhh a doctor
30        who's gonna see her this morning ((continues))
```

(Beach, 2001, pp. 232–33, adapted)

Perhaps the most striking thing about this conversation is how the 'good news' of the mother's stabilizing condition takes on an ambiguous status in the context of the son's lifeworld, in which things like work commitments, airline schedules and ticket prices impinge on the way he is able to take action around his mother's illness. Reframed within this web of personal and professional pressures, the discussion of his mother's health becomes a calculative assessment regarding how long his mother has to live versus how long he can afford to be away from work. Ironically, the primary risk the son faces as he makes his travel plans is not that his mother will die, but that she *won't* die during his visit and that he will have to disrupt his work schedule again at a later date. This is not to imply that the son is unfeeling. Rather, it is meant to highlight how health-related events have a way of rupturing the 'obdurate orderliness' of everyday life (Maynard, 1996, p. 4), complicating mundane concerns about things like work, school, shopping, and traffic, which, while not matters of 'life and death', still carry their own urgency. Often these other concerns function to reframe discussions about health and risk, and sometimes discussions about these concerns become tools which people use to talk about health and risk when talking about them directly is difficult, awkward, or emotionally upsetting.

The couple in this transcript are not only using the son's travel plans to talk about the mother's health – they are also using the mother's health to talk about their own relationship. In other words, 'mom's cancer' has become a tool with which this recently divorced couple negotiates their own intimacy and the ex-wife's ambiguous status within the family. G begins the conversation by using the occasion of mom's cancer as an opportunity to reaffirm intimacy ('I lov:e yo:u: … I wanted to *tell* you tha:t = '). The son, however, while treating his ex-wife as having the rights of a family member in being updated about his mother's condition, seems to take pains to create distance between them by answering her profession of love with a dispreferred response ('thanks'), and deploying frustration about his mother's condition and his travel plans to pre-empt any further displays of affection; in saying that he thought G's phone call was actually news about his mother's condition, for example, he provides for himself a warrant to end the call sooner than might normally be expected. In fact, Beach notes similar features in other conversations between S and G in the course of making plans around the mother's illness and notes how, through the iterative delivery of news about 'mom's cancer', this couple manages their 'close yet estranged relationship as a recently divorced couple remaining in "friendly" contact' (2001, p. 243).

Dinnertime conversations

Another example of how discussions of health within families function as tools for the negotiation of intimacy and power can be seen in Paugh and Izquierdo's (2009) study of dinnertime conversations between parents and children in which parents try to socialize their children into healthy eating habits. Struggles between parents and children over health-related practices are an extremely rich site of investigation, not just because they can reveal how issues of family dynamics can affect health behavior, but also because they are where children learn practices of communication around health and risk that they carry into their later lives.

The example below is an excerpt from a longer interaction in which parents Alice and Tommy attempt to limit the food consumption of their nine-year-old daughter Linda while also struggling to manage the behavior of her younger brother, Daniel. The parents are extremely concerned about their daughter's eating habits and have enrolled her in a pediatric weight management program. In discussions with the researchers, both Alice and Tommy framed Linda's problem as a 'lack of self-control'. 'She can't control her diet,' her father explained. 'She just eats the wrong foods. She doesn't seem to care about what she eats or how she looks' (p. 194). The excerpt below occurs near the end of a meal in which Linda and her parents have already engaged in a long, drawn-out negotiation about how much she should be allowed to eat.

27	Linda:	Tell him he can't have seconds 'cause =
28	Daniel:	[((returns to table and drops a handful of French fries on his plate))
29	Linda:	[= ((sees Daniel and starts yelling)) THAT'S NOT FAIR THAT HE GETS ALL THE FRIES!
30	Tommy:	Linda, you have plenty.
31	Daniel:	There's only a little-[can I have the REST?
32	Linda:	[NO I DIDN'T!
33	Linda:	I'M STILL HUNGRY HERE!
34	Daniel:	((pointing toward the kitchen)) Mom can I have the rest?
35	Linda:	'Cause I didn't have that much =
36	Daniel:	Mom can I have the rest of (the fries)?
37	Alice:	((shakes head once and then cocks it from side to side as if unsure))
38	Linda:	[= for lunch.
39	Daniel:	[((running to the kitchen)) I'll take (xxx)
40	Linda:	I just had soup
41	Daniel:	((from kitchen)) Mom there's only one.
42	Alice:	((to Linda)) What do you want extra of?
43	Linda:	I don't know pasta [(xxx)
44	Alice:	[Maybe some peas and carrots
45	Daniel:	((returns to the table with something in his hand, does not sit but begins eating))
46	Tommy:	((calmly, to Linda)) Would you like a turkey meatball?
47	Linda:	((quietly)) Can I have both? Pasta and a little bit of turkey meatball?
48	Tommy:	((takes a meatball from his plate and passes it to Linda))
49	Alice:	((jumps up quickly and goes to kitchen)) I'll make some- I'm going to warm up some more pasta.
50	Tommy:	((to Linda)) You're welcome [re: for the meatball]
51	Linda:	Thank you.
52	Alice:	Tommy I'll give her a little bit more pasta
53	Daniel:	I want pasta mommy.
54	Linda:	You got fries DANIEL! That should be enough for you 'cause you got FRIES.
55	Alice:	Linda you know what [(xxx).
56	Tommy:	[Linda, worry about yourself.
57	Daniel:	((leaning toward Linda, speaking mockingly)) You (xxxx).
58	Linda:	((shoves Daniel back toward his seat))

(Paugh and Izquierdo, 2009, pp. 196–97)

Despite the parents' best intentions at limiting their daughter's intake of food, Linda manages in this excerpt (as she apparently has on many other occasions) to get her own way, securing for herself not just a hamburger (already given to her at a previous point in the transcript), but also a turkey meatball and some pasta. She does this by strategically reframing the conversation from one about health and diet to one about parental fairness and sibling equality. By doing this, she usurps the 'moral high ground' from her parents, who originally try to make the conversation about Linda and her lack of 'self-control'.

This example suggests that, rather than solely a matter of her lack of 'self-control', Linda's eating habits are also a consequence of her parents' behavior towards her. Their part in Linda's overeating is not just the fact that they give into her, but *how* they give in. Tommy, for example, does not verbally respond to her demands, but nevertheless responds by giving her a meatball from his plate, and then himself reframes the exchange from a lesson about diet to one about politeness, saying 'you're welcome' (line 50) to prompt Linda to say 'thank you'. Meanwhile, Alice, appearing to take this as a signal that they have lost the battle, goes into the kitchen to prepare more pasta for Linda. By the end of the excerpt, the locus of the interaction has shifted almost completely away from food to the behavior of the two children towards each other and of the parents towards them (which, after all, is what Linda has wanted all along).

I include this example not just to demonstrate how easily a nine-year-old girl can manipulate her parents using the strategies of framing and positioning I outlined in the last chapter, but also to show how individual health behavior in such contexts is rarely just a matter of individual character or 'will-power', but is also a matter of the patterns of social interaction in which such behavior develops and plays out. Although in interviews the two parents in this example expressed the strong desire to help Linda learn to regulate her diet, in actual interactions with her at mealtimes what they actually end up doing is helping her to hone her negotiation skills. By allowing her to challenge them repeatedly and then giving in, they socialize her (and her brother) in how to 'engage in conflict and negotiation over food' (see also Ochs and Shohet, 2006; p. 197).

Risky interactions

Perhaps the greatest unanswered question of health communication is why people continue to put themselves at risk despite having access to knowledge and other resources for risk reduction. People who smoke, have unsafe sex with strangers, take dangerous drugs, and engage in a host of other obviously risky behaviors are often thought of as behaving 'irrationally'. This judgment is based on a model of human behavior which conceives of the social actor as an autonomous individual who can be counted on to make rational decisions based on the available knowledge, and so health promotion efforts based on this model generally begin with the assumption that people take risks either because they lack the requisite knowledge or they hold some attitudes or beliefs that make it difficult to 'put that knowledge into practice'. The whole notion of 'putting knowledge into practice', in fact, sums up the epistemological position of this approach.

It is not hard to see the limitations of this model in understanding the kinds of risk-taking illustrated in the vignettes with which I began this chapter, both of which involve not just the simple application of knowledge to decision-making, but also involve complex social relationships and social contexts. In fact, most risk behavior is *not* purely a matter of 'rational' decision-making by autonomous social actors, but rather a 'socially interactive enterprise' (Rhodes, 1997, p. 211) which is invariably affected by a host of factors like the relative power and social status of participants. Whatever the role played by deliberative decision-making in risk behavior, it is clear from experience that more knowledge does not necessarily translate into 'better' decisions, and the abstract rationality of health promoters is not always the same as the 'situated rationality' of actual social actors (Bloor, 1995; Parsons and Atkinson, 1992).

Another way of understanding risk behavior has been to go to the opposite extreme: rather than focusing on the rational individual, focusing instead on the behavior of large populations and identifying the 'factors' by which certain groups can be identified as 'at risk'. This more epidemiological approach to risk behavior grew out of the large-scale studies of health behavior in populations that gained currency in the 1950s and 1960s, the most famous being the Framingham Heart Study initiated in 1948, which dramatically changed the way doctors thought about and treated heart disease. It was, in fact, in the Framingham Heart Study that the term 'risk factor' was coined (Kannel et al., 1962).

Although the simple definition of a 'risk factor' is any variable that puts people at a higher risk for contracting or developing a disease or condition, what actually constitutes a risk factor is quite complicated. Risk factors may involve behavior such as smoking, may involve characteristics that have little to do with behavior like membership in a particular social or ethnic group, or may involve external environmental factors over which people have little or no control (Rothstein, 2003). What makes something a 'risk factor' is not necessarily that it has any direct role in 'causing' risk, but that it is *associated* with higher risk from a statistical point of view. This is what makes the concept of the risk factor both such a powerful tool for epidemiologists and actuaries, and often such a difficult tool for clinicians and health promoters to put to practical use, for, while such factors have predictive power, they lack *explanatory* power (Berg and Grimes, 2011). Focusing on 'risk factors' to understand behavior also tends to obscure the role of individual agency as it unfolds over the course of a particular event or series of events. While the 'rational actor' model discussed above relies perhaps too much on assumptions of individual agency, in population-based models, actors are often seen as more or less at the mercy of their demographic characteristics, their environments, or their behaviors, which are often treated more as attributes than as agentive choices.

Applied linguistics makes available a number of analytical tools that can help us avoid the extremes of methodological individualism that characterize the 'rational actor' model and the methodological collectivism that characterizes population-based approaches, tools which allow us to analyze risk as it actually unfolds in situated interactions as people discursively manage 'what they are doing' and 'who they are being'. It is a perspective that shifts our attention to the ways 'real' people in 'real' sites of engagement accomplish actions by drawing on the discursive resources available to them.

One challenge in studying such sites of engagement is that many of them are not as readily accessible to researchers as dinnertime conversations or phone calls between relatives because they involve intensely private and sometimes illegal activities like sex and drug use. Thus, rather than relying on detailed transcripts like those presented above and in the previous chapter, we are forced to 'piece together' these 'risky interactions' by analyzing people's accounts of them. This, of course, invariably complicates our analysis since accounts are themselves socially occasioned actions which are affected by such factors as the people to whom the accounting is made, and the perceived purpose of the account. The way someone accounts for risky behavior is likely to be different if he or she is giving the account to a spouse, a doctor, a police officer or a researcher.

Many sociological studies of risk using qualitative data focus only on the 'content' of such accounts, treating participants' reports of events as unproblematic reflections of their actions and intentions. Applied linguists, on the other hand, are more accustomed to seeing accounts as 'versions of reality' and to focusing on the strategies of entextualization people use to highlight certain aspects of their experience and background others. The purpose of such analysis is not so much to understand what 'really happened' as it is to understand how people understand, organize, and reconstruct the 'orderliness' of what happened in ways that make themselves 'accountable' as competent members of the social groups to which they belong. Despite their inevitably subjective nature, people's accounts of their risky behaviors have considerable advantages over the questionnaire surveys that form the basis of epidemiological approaches to risk, which suffer from the same limitations as other self-report data but usually lack the ability to capture details about the 'processural' (Rhodes, 1997) nature of episodes of risk-taking from the participants' point of view.

There are a variety of frameworks within applied linguistics for analyzing people's accounts of their actions, from narrative analysis (Riessman, 1993) to discursive psychology (Edwards and Potter, 1992). Here I will focus on three broad aspects of such accounts that seem particularly relevant for understanding risk: (1) the way people use such accounts to show their 'competence' as members of their social groups; (2) the way people use such accounts to explain or justify their motives and assign agency to various people, objects, or circumstances; and (3) the way people represent the concrete actions which they and others took during the encounter and arrange those actions as parts of sequential chains of action and as parts of larger activities or social practices. I will discuss these three aspects under the headings of *the grammar of context*, *the grammar of motives*, and *the grammar of action*.

The grammar of context

Most risk-taking takes place in the context of specific kinds of speech events which occur in specific kinds of places, and a large part of the way people organize and understand their risk-taking has to do with their expectations of how these speech events themselves are organized. Just as people bring to medical consultations certain preconceived ideas about who will say or do what to whom, when, where and how, they bring similar sets of 'rules' to situations in which they might engage in risky behavior, such as parties, skateboarding sessions, or visits to public sex venues.

Scollon and his colleagues (2012) use the term 'grammar of context' to describe the sets of expectations shared by members of particular communities regarding how certain recognizable speech events ought to be carried out, including where, when, and why they should occur. Their outline for the grammar of context is based on Hymes' SPEAKING model, which forms the basis of the ethnography of communication (Gumperz and Hymes, 1964; Hymes, 1974). For Hymes, one's 'communicative competence' based on one's mastery of the 'grammar of context' is every bit as important as one's linguistic competence in demonstrating that one is a legitimate member of a speech community. At the same time, like language grammars, context grammars are dynamic and flexible, with people 'breaking rules' and producing 'marked forms' strategically in order to create certain kinds of socially situated meanings.

The seven components of the grammar of context Scollon and his colleagues propose are *setting* (including time, place, location, and use of space), *key* (the 'mood' or level of formality associated with the speech event), *participants* (including expectations about participant roles and rights), *message form* (the mode and media of communication participants use), *sequence* (referring both to the overall sequencing of actions and to more micro-level sequencing of utterances into adjacency pairs), *co-occurrence patterns* (the features of the interactions which are likely to occur together), and *manifestation* (the degree to which the 'rules' of the grammar of context are implicit or explicit).

The way people account for risk behavior can often reveal a great deal about their underlying assumptions about the speech events within which these risky actions occur and how they fit into community norms and practices. Such understanding is particularly important for health promoters who wish to design targeted interventions for particular groups. Health promoters who provide condoms and safe sex information in public sex venues, for example, must understand the norms of communication that members adhere to in such venues so that they can 'fit in' (see for example Jones, 2002b). For participants themselves, talk of 'what we do' is a way of both enacting identity within a particular community and of locating responsibility for their individual risk-taking in community norms.

A good example of a study in which participants' accounts are analyzed to reconstruct the 'grammar of context' which governs the circumstances in which risk-taking takes place is Eggert and Nicholas' (1992) ethnography of teenage truancy and drug use in a suburban high school. For Eggert and Nicholas, 'skippin'' and 'gettin' high' are 'rule-based' speech events in which participants share sets of expectations about things like setting, participant roles, and 'ways of speaking'. 'Skippin'', for example, is described by participants as taking place in certain set locations, each associated with different times of day, different specific activities, and even different kinds of 'skippers'. Similarly, 'gettin' high' is not just about taking drugs (chiefly cannabis), but also involves complex codes of friendship and reciprocity around buying and sharing drugs. To be accepted by the group, for example, members are expected to smoke and drink as much as others – smoking or drinking too little or too much may be cause for comment. Members are also expected to share drugs and alcohol freely with other members, based on a tacit system of reciprocity, and when they do not do so they risk social sanction.

Perhaps the most interesting finding of Eggert and Nicholas's study is that many of the students who engage in the activities of 'skippin'' and 'gettin' high' are not non-conformists or even poor students, and much of what characterizes these activities is not a 'lack of discipline' (as their teachers and parents contend), but rather a particularly strongly developed set of norms about the importance of maintaining discipline and self-control. Eggert and Nicholas compare 'skippin'' to a game, and summarize the strategies of competent players as follows:

(1) Use common sense about how much to skip (the 'common sense' or good judgment and caution rule).
(2) Keep skippin' and gettin' high low-key (the 'keep it quiet' or covert rule).
(3) Keep track of or keep a running record of skips (the 'maintaining control' or monitoring rule).
(4) Take care to cover skips with creative notes, phone calls, and prearranged absences; tell a good story and provide acceptable or compelling excuses for absences (the 'following the teacher's rule' or 'working the system' rule).
(5) Get in as many skips as possible but still pass the class and graduate (the 'skippin' but still graduating' or 'having your cake and eating it too' rule).

(p. 83)

While those participants in the study who position themselves as 'smart skippers' value having a 'good time' (which includes the 'thrill' of risk-taking), they also value 'judgment' and 'common sense'. In fact, part of the 'good time' for them involves 'testing their limits' and exercising their calculative and imaginative faculties. One participant, for example, makes a point of recording all of her 'skips' in an appointment book. 'I don't know if I'm weird or not,' she says, 'but I just keep track of my skips and who I skip with … an' of the number of times I get high. That way I don't always miss the same class.' At the same time, students who do not exercise discipline and self-control are considered 'bad skippers' whose behavior not only hurts themselves but also increases the risks for the group as a whole:

They're not playing the game right … They're doing it right out in the open … they probably don't care if people notice! Gettin' high everyday – usually in the morning before school, at lunch, and again at the end of the school day, that's usin' too much … it could get you into trouble.

(p. 84)

What this and studies like it reveal is that while risk-taking might seem illogical to people outside of communities of risk-takers, the social occasions in which risk-taking takes place are often governed by their own 'local logic'. This logic often involves rules about social relationships (e.g. 'fairness' and 'loyalty'), which sometimes override concerns about health or safety. They also highlight the fact that risk-takers often see their behavior not just in the context of particular social groups and particular speech events, but also as embedded in the 'ecology' of their broader social worlds, which includes the demands of school, work, family obligations, and the constraints placed on them by authority figures.

The grammar of motives

As I discussed above, much health promotion discourse regarding things like drug abuse and unsafe sex is predicated on locating *agency* in the minds of the social actors. Individuals are seen to be responsible for their own actions and enough in control of their fate to avoid circumstances (and people) that might make it more difficult for them to act rationally. As I discussed in chapter 3, however, the way agency is constructed in health-related texts is sometimes ambiguous, subject to various ideological or institutional agendas. As van Leeuwen (1996) points out, there is rarely a neat fit between grammatical agency and the actual degree to which different social actors are really able to exercise control in 'real life' situations. This is because, while entextualizations are always partial, 'real life' situations are complicated. It is usually impossible to assign agency for social actions to one person or thing or another. Rather, agency is *distributed* across people, settings, texts, and other artifacts. When I cross a busy urban street, I cannot do so alone. I depend on the other people crossing the street with me, the people driving cars and lorries, the government officials who have drafted the regulations and created the signs, traffic lights and pavement markings that make crossing the street safe, as well as various officers of the law who enforce these regulations to make 'my' crossing of the street possible.

The point I'm trying to make is that risk-taking is always to some extent a matter of 'shared responsibility': partly dependent on the thoughts and intentions of the individual, partly dependent on other people with whom he or she is acting, partly dependent on the circumstances in which the interaction takes place and the availability of various resources for engaging in or avoiding risk behavior, and partly dependent on community and institutional rules and norms (the 'grammar of context') that govern how different people are expected to act in the situation. When people account for their actions in retrospect, they are always faced with the task of *framing* those actions and *positioning* themselves in relation to them in ways that rhetorically assign responsibility to one or more aspects of the situation, whether it be their own intentions, the actions of the people with whom they were acting, or the environment or circumstances in which the actions took place.

In his influential book, *A Grammar of Motives*, Kenneth Burke (1969) argues that when people talk about their reasons for doing things, they tend to organize their accounts based on five distinct 'perspectives': the perspective of the *social actor* and his or her own 'will' or motivation (which Burke calls the 'agent'), the perspective of the '*scene*' in which the action occurs, including the physical, social, and cultural

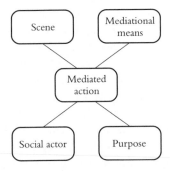

FIGURE 5.1 Burke's pentad of motives, adapted from Scollon and Scollon (2004, p. 127)

circumstances in which the action takes place, the perspective of the *mediational means* (such as texts and other artifacts) that the actor has available to him or her to take the action (what Burke calls the 'agency'), the perspective of the 'purpose' of the action and its expected outcomes, and the perspective of the action itself (what Burke calls the 'act') with its own force of 'momentum'. In many accounts, agency is distributed strategically across perspectives as the story progresses. Scollon and Scollon summarize Burke's 'pentad of motives' in the diagram reprinted in Figure 5.1.

Burke's interest was not to discover 'what really happened' in the events that people are recounting, but rather to come up with a framework with which to analyze the way people make themselves accountable for their actions by discursively locating agency in different aspects of the situation. Similarly, the goal of the applied linguistic approach I have been developing here is not to somehow find out 'who is to blame' for risky behavior, but rather to understand how people discursively construct their risky actions and position themselves in relation to them.

A number of qualitative studies of sexual risk and HIV/AIDS have yielded a rich collection of accounts of unsafe sex from a variety of different kinds of people including heterosexual women (Sobo, 1995), gay men (Jones and Candlin, 2003; Mutchler, 2000), teenagers (Harrison, Xaba, and Kunene, 2001), and people living with HIV (Cusick and Rhodes, 2002). While few of these studies make explicit use of Burke's grammar of motives, many attempt to explain the mechanisms through which storytellers frame their accounts and position themselves in them as more or less responsible for their actions.

Among the most important aspects of the way people account for risk-taking, as Cusick and Rhodes (2002) point out, is whether they frame what occurred with reference to normative ideas about safety and risk (for example, 'use a condom every time'), or whether they attempt to frame what happened in terms of some alternative framework of safety and risk. Based on their analysis of seventy-three accounts of unsafe sex from HIV+ men and women, collected in London in the late 1990s, they note that those who frame their accounts in terms of normative models of 'safe sex' are more likely to account for episodes of unsafe sex by locating agency outside of the self, in other people ('he wouldn't take no for an answer'), in the mediational means ('the condom broke'), or in the circumstances in which the unsafe sex took place ('we were drunk/high', 'we didn't have a condom'). Those who are willing to take either individual or collective (with their partner) responsibility for their actions, on the other hand, often justify them by attempting to *reframe* notions of safe sex, to, in effect, redefine safety, or even to question it as a value altogether. Typically such reframings in their data occurred in instances in which participants were having sex with partners they knew (or assumed) to be HIV+ as well, a circumstance in which they believed that the 'rules' of safe sex did not apply. Other participants in the study redefined risk by assigning agency to the purpose of the encounter, with goals like the expression of love and commitment trumping goals of safety. One participant with an HIV+ partner put it this way:

> We both knew we loved each other very much. We just agreed we would do it [dispense with condoms] and it might sound crazy to an awful lot of people out there, but we really believed absolutely because of how we felt about each other just total unconditional love for each other.
>
> *(Cusick and Rhodes, 2002, p. 202)*

This example illustrates that acts of risk-taking themselves are acts of positioning, means by which people claim various identities for themselves and impute identities to their partners. Countless studies have shown that many people regard unprotected sex as a means of expressing love, trust, or commitment (see for example Jones et al., 2000; Keogh et al., 1998; Rosenthal et al., 1998; Sobo, 1995). Of course, the flip-side of this is that using condoms can have the effect of claiming and imputing 'spoiled identities' (Goffman, 1963). As one participant in a study I conducted of AIDS-related communication among gay men in China (Jones, 2002a, 2007) described it:

> If I like my partner … it feels strange to use this [a condom] … it gives the feeling that you don't trust me … you think I'm dirty … and if you reverse it … no … you're not dirty … I just want to protect you … then I'm dirty … this is the most important reason.
>
> *(Jones, 2007, p. 107)*

Another example of strategic reframing can be seen in the accounts of those who engage in 'bareback sex' (see for example Adam, 2005, 2006), who, like the 'skippers' described above, often frame their activities not in terms of pleasure and abandon, but rather in terms of responsibility and control. In many communities where 'barebacking' is regularly practiced, it is accompanied by careful processes of 'sero-sorting' (determining the probable HIV status of all involved) and strong values placed on communication and honesty. In fact, as Adam (2005) points out, much discourse on 'barebacking' frames the activity squarely within normative health promotion discourses of 'personal responsibility' and 'informed consent' along with neo-liberal values of 'free choice'. As one of the HIV+ participants in Cusick and Rhodes's study put it:

While I do believe that I have a responsibility not to infect people I think the ultimate responsibility has to be for yourself. Ultimately it has to be an individual's responsibility.

(Cusick and Rhodes, 2002, p. 221)

The grammar of action

As I mentioned above, some people, when accounting for risk behavior, locate the motivation for the behavior not in themselves, in the circumstances, or in the purpose of the behavior, but rather in the sense of 'momentum' associated with the behavior itself. Individuals, for example, may plan to refrain from unsafe sex or initiate sexual contact with the intention of using a condom, only to be swept up in the chain of actions that constitutes the sexual act. People often describe this phenomenon with expressions like 'one thing led to another', portraying actions themselves as having their own 'agency' independent of the conscious control of social actors.

Whereas the *grammar of context* explores how people construct the contextual rules of speech events (who says what to whom, when, where, and how), and the *grammar of motives* explores how people frame accounts of risk and position them-selves within them in ways that locate agency in different aspects of the situation, the *grammar of action* seeks to identify patterns in the way people describe the actual actions that they and the people with whom they were acting took, and how these actions are linked together and organized in narratives.

A focus on actions, rather than just on the motives people assign to those actions, helps us to attend to the dynamic and *procedural* nature of risk behavior and serves as an antidote to naïve assumptions that people are always conscious of why they do things. At the same time, understanding how people organize past actions can give us important insights into how they anticipate and plan for future ones.

In the last chapter I discussed how framing in medical encounters can be understood in terms of *sequentiality* and *simultaneity*. What I mean by sequentiality is the fact that interactions move forward in stages in which the accomplishment of one stage lays the groundwork for the initiation of the next stage, and, within stages, exchanges are organized in sequences whose parts are linked together in relationships of 'conditional relevance' (Sacks, 1967; Schegloff, 1968), in which one utterance both creates a 'slot' for the next utterance and provides evidence regarding how the previous utterance was understood. I also pointed out how, in actual interactions, participants often violate or defy this sequential order for strategic reasons, and that what makes such violations meaningful or strategically effective is the underlying assumption people bring to interactions that they will be conducted in an orderly manner.

What I mean by simultaneity is that, at any given moment many actions are invariably being performed at the same time, these different actions often occurring on different 'timescales'. A moment in which a couple decides to dispense with a condom is embedded in a longer episode of 'having sex', which is embedded in an

evening's activities (a 'date', for example), which is embedded in a longer relationship, which is embedded in the longer sexual careers of those involved. Just as
clients of genetic counselors understand the risk of developing or passing on certain
genetically determined conditions differently depending on the 'timeframe' in
which the risk is presented, so do individuals who engage in risky behavior like
unsafe sex understand the risk differently depending on whether they see their
actions as part of a one-off sexual encounter or whether they see them as part of a
longer-term relationship with the other person. In the last chapter I called processes
through which people 'scale up' or 'scale down' their temporal perspectives on
their actions 'circumferencing' (Scollon and Scollon, 2004).

Despite the apparent spontaneity associated with risk-taking behavior, people
bring to it the same kind of expectations about the 'orderliness' of human interaction, and interpret what they are doing using the same processes of 'circumferencing' that they do in more formal interactions, and when they talk about such
behavior they often attempt to recreate that orderliness in their accounts. When
talking about episodes of unsafe sex, for example, people often arrange the actions
in their narratives in a way that each action is portrayed as creating the conditions for
or 'inviting' subsequent actions, and providing evidence as to how previous actions
have been interpreted by partners.

Figure 5.2, for example, is an excerpt from a diary entry from a gay man talking
about an episode of unsafe sex (Jones and Candlin, 2003, p. 206). In the excerpt I
have arranged the actions in a way that illustrates the way the narrator assigns
agency at different moments in the encounter.

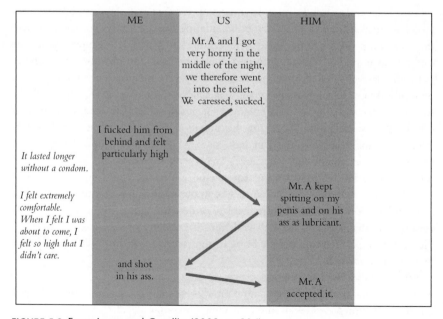

FIGURE 5.2 From Jones and Candlin (2003, p. 206)

Analysis of such an account from the perspective of the *grammar of motives* would focus more on the 'commentary' of events given by the storyteller (arranged in Figure 5.2 in the far left column), noting how he locates responsibility for his actions in his own inability to control himself ('I felt so high that I didn't care'). Such an analysis alone, however, would fail to take into account the way agency is constructed in the portrayal of the actions themselves, with the actions the narrator took presented as 'responding to' his partner's actions and 'inviting' responses from him. In this way he presents the incident as both cooperatively constructed and, in a sense, 'orderly' – despite his admission of loss of control.

Two important points arise from this example. The first is the way actions themselves are taken to have meaning, and the processes of implicature and inference that go into the production of this meaning. Despite the advice in public health discourse to 'talk about safe sex', most negotiation of sexual contact (as well as many other potentially 'risky' activities) is largely silent (conducted through actions, facial expression and other non-verbal behaviour) and heavily context dependent. In different communities and different contexts, certain actions are taken to have meanings, whether or not these meanings are actually intended by the people who took these actions. In Cusick and Rhodes's (2002) study of accounts of unsafe sex by HIV+ individuals, a number of the interviewees indicated that when their partners did not explicitly suggest that they use condoms, they took this as a signal that that person must be HIV+ themselves. Such appeals take unprotected sex itself as an implication of positive status and as a warrant for continued unprotected sex. As one of their participants put it:

> God, you know, if a guy is twenty-eight or thirty, they know. If they are willing to just go ahead without a condom, then I assume that they must be [positive].
> *(Cusick and Rhodes, 2002, p. 222)*

The second important point to note in the above example is the way agency alternates between parties. It is not so much that agency is 'shared' or distributed as it is that it is 'traded' in a kind of back-and-forth manner. The reason this observation is important is that it shows how sometimes assigning responsibility for risk is not as straightforward as it might seem. In many situations in which risk is negotiated, agency is dynamically claimed and imputed by different parties at different times as the interaction progresses.

Just as accounts of unsafe sex are often organized as 'orderly' chains of actions, they also often present risk behavior in the context of broader socially recognized activities or social practices occurring on different timescales. The way risky actions are portrayed depends a great deal on how we 'frame' them – what we say we are 'doing' when we are having sex. In the following excerpt, an episode of unsafe sex is framed in terms of a long-term relationship between the narrator and his lover.

> When we were seized with a sudden impulse to have sex, I asked him not to use a condom in order to have a more intimate contact and he agreed.

> When he inserted his cock into my ass our sex and love were more sub-
> stantial. Compared with using a condom, you can feel that sex without a
> condom is more exciting. Exempted from the worry of AIDS, sex is more
> enjoyable and exciting. ... In fact, under such romantic conditions, you
> really don't think about AIDS. Instead, you feel safe to have sex with him
> because you believe that he is faithful to you.
>
> *(Jones and Candlin, 2003, p. 207)*

In this example, the chain of actions leading up to the risk-taking on the shorter
timescale of the actual encounter (the request for unsafe sex, the assent, the pene-
tration of one partner by another) is framed within a longer timescale activity, the
relationship between two parties, a relationship which is portrayed as having
developed to a point where safer sex has become a barrier to intimacy. Observed
from the vantage point of this timescale, unsafe sex is portrayed as a 'natural' outcome of a longer process. The story of risk told along the shorter timescale of the
encounter is subordinated to the story of 'love' told along the longer timescale of
the relationship. At the same time, this 'love story', with its trajectory leading
inevitably towards risk behavior, is portrayed not just as *their* story, but as *the* story
of love. The narrator accomplishes this portrayal by strategically shifting pronouns
from 'I/we' in the beginning of the account ('I asked him not to use a condom') to
'you' ('you feel safe to have sex with him') towards the end. The primary function
of 'you' here is to transform the individual experience of the narrator into a
universal one by invoking a 'cultural storyline' with its own prototypical trajectory
which links the narrator and his partner to the larger community and culture of
which they are a part. Such invocations of both longer-scale perspectives and cultural storylines is a common feature of accounts of risk across a variety of contexts
(see for example Plumridge and Chetwynd, 1999).

One interesting aspect of the example above is that despite the fact that the decision
to engage in unsafe sex is the result of explicit sexual negotiation, which, ironically,
conforms to advice from health promoters to 'talk about unsafe sex' ('I asked him not
to use a condom ... and he agreed'), the narrator nevertheless uses the language of
inevitability and loss of control to describe the act itself ('when we were seized
with a sudden impulse ... ', 'In fact, under such romantic conditions, you really
don't think about AIDS'). That is to say, while on the one hand the action is
portrayed as 'deliberative', on the other hand it is portrayed as having its own
momentum – a sense that 'under such romantic conditions', there is 'no turning
back'. This sense of 'no turning back' also extends beyond this episode, after which
the narrator finds not using a condom with his partner much easier. At the same
time, not using condoms seems to decrease rather than increase the narrator's
anxiety about HIV infection – unsafe sex, when reframed as long-term love and
commitment, has the effect of 'exempting' the couple from 'the worry of AIDS'.

Scollon (2001b) calls this sense of momentum or 'inevitability' that develops in
certain social situations the 'funnel of commitment'. What he means by this is that
the sequentiality of the actions we engage in and their simultaneous enactment of

longer-scale storylines play a role in our ability to resist or interrupt chains of actions. As I mentioned in chapter 2, to illustrate this concept Scollon gives the example of buying a cup of coffee, noting that the further along we progress in this chain of actions – entering the coffee shop, choosing a product, placing our order, paying, and accepting the coffee from the server – the harder it becomes to change or reverse this chain of actions. This is because of the dual 'force' of the *syntagmatic* (sequential) and the *paradigmatic* (simultaneous) dimensions of the activity, the syntagmatic dimension driving the activity forward through the power of one action to create the conditions for the next, and the paradigmatic dimension driving the actions forward by virtue of the expectations participants share about what should happen based on the longer timescale activities or 'cultural storylines' that they see the actions to be part of.

From this perspective, rather than asking why a particular individual did or did not use a condom in a particular sexual encounter we might more productively ask: At what points in this encounter did using a condom become either more or less 'possible', and how was this affected by partners' shared expectations about how 'one thing follows another' in certain kinds of sexual encounters and certain kinds of relationships? The value of this way of thinking is that it gives researchers, counselors, and those who engage in risk behavior themselves a way to analyze what happened that avoids the fatalism implied in narratives of lost control ('I just couldn't help myself') and the self-blame implied in narratives of personal responsibility ('I should have known better').

*

In this and previous chapters I have outlined some of the basic analytical principles that form the foundation of an applied linguistic approach to health and risk communication. I have shown how different 'versions' of health and risk are constructed in texts through the use of various linguistic resources, and how both professionals and laypeople appropriate these notions of health and risk in specific 'sites of engagement' in order to enact various social practices and claim and impute social identities. In the next two chapters I will make use of these principles to explore a kind of entextualization that is particularly central to communication about health and risk – the entextualization of the human body.

6

HEALTH, RISK, AND THE ENTEXTUALIZED BODY

In 1994 John Baldetta, a nurse's aide in Seattle's Harborview Medical Centre, was fired for refusing to cover up a tattoo on his inner left forearm of the words 'HIV Positive'. Baldetta sued the hospital for violating his right to free speech and discriminating against him on the basis of his disability. 'I'm being treated like a disease, not a person,' he told the press.

Baldetta said that he got the tattoo in order to help raise awareness about HIV and dispel the stigma attached to it, but the hospital contended that it was not his job to educate people. The United States Court of Appeals agreed with the hospital, denying Baldetta's claims of disability discrimination, reasoning that he had been excluded from his position not because of being HIV positive, but because of his tattoo, which was a text that he had produced volitionally rather than an unavoidable manifestation of his illness. Similarly, the court found that Baldetta's rights to free speech were not violated by the prohibition on displaying the tattoo since its display in the context of a hospital ward could be regarded as 'disruptive'. At the same time, the court found that the hospital's prohibition on Baldetta *talking* about HIV with patients *did* constitute a possible violation of his right to free speech. In other words, he could not be prohibited from talking about HIV, but he could be prohibited from making his body a text upon which others could read his HIV positive status (Bassett, 2012).

Around the same time, the Italian sportswear company Benetton released an ad campaign featuring pictures of models bearing tattoos that read 'HIV Positive'. As with Baldetta's tattoo, the case of Benetton's HIV tattoo ad campaign ended up in court. In a French court Benetton was fined US$32,000 in a case brought against it by three HIV positive people and the AIDES Federation Nationale, the court finding that the campaign was an abuse of free speech and a 'provocative exploitation of suffering' (Campos,

2011). The reason the company's director of communications Peter Fressola gave for displaying these tattoos, was not that different from the one given by Baldetta for displaying his: to raise awareness about HIV. 'There are a lot of people who believe the greatest foe in the fight against AIDS is invisibility,' he said. 'These ads are designed [to] raise awareness of a serious issue, to make awareness our label' (Spindler, 1993).

Today a growing number of HIV positive people wear tattoos depicting the biohazard symbol to advertise their sero-status (Figure 6.1). Many do so in the same spirit of Baldetta and Fressola, in order to 'raise awareness' about HIV and combat the sense of shame often associated with the disease. One man with such a tattoo is quoted in a news report (Landau, 2011) as saying: 'It's a branding of who I am, and it's a branding of being comfortable with that.' For some, however, these tattoos also have a more practical function: in the subcultural practice of 'barebacking' – intentional unsafe sex – they provide a way for HIV negative men who are turned on by risky sex (called 'bugchasers') to identify potential HIV positive partners (Poland and Holmes, 2009; Shernoff, 2006).

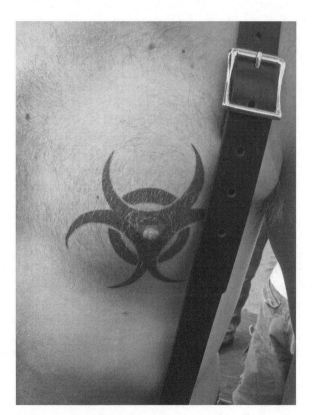

FIGURE 6.1 Biohazard tattoo: istolethetv, available for use under the Creative Commons license

*

In chapter 3 I discussed how social practices and social identities associated with health and risk are 'technologized' in texts like health promotion pamphlets, medical case reports, and newspaper stories, and in the last two chapters I focused on how these practices and identities are negotiated in social interactions through strategies of framing and positioning. In this chapter and the next I will consider what happens when the body itself is transformed into a text and the different kinds of social actions around health and risk that people can take using these texts.

The three examples above illustrate some of the issues associated with entextualizations of the body, which I will develop. The first has to do with the status of the entextualized body as a *mediational means* with which to take social action. What is striking about the examples that I discussed above is that essentially the same text – a tattoo disclosing HIV status – can be used to take so many different kinds of actions, actions such as fighting discrimination, creating awareness, challenging one's boss, engaging in unsafe sex, defending oneself in a court of law, or selling knitwear.

The second issue these examples illustrate is the way textual bodies exist in complex webs of intertextuality and interdiscursivity. The potential for these texts to make possible the kinds of actions discussed above depends on their being read in relation to a host of other texts that have become part of the 'archive' of our experience with disease and stigma: texts like the yellow stars and pink triangles that were used by the Nazis to brand Jews and homosexuals, texts like newspaper articles such as that written by conservative columnist William Buckley in the 1980s suggesting that 'Everyone detected with AIDS should be tattooed in the upper forearm and on the buttocks' (Buckley, 1986), and various legal texts like the Americans with Disabilities Act. Textual bodies, once they are created, also go on to form new intertextual links with yet other texts, in this case letters of dismissal, legal briefs, court decisions, and even chapters in books about applied linguistic approaches to health communication.

The third important issue is the fact that how these entextualized bodies are used also depends crucially on who controls them: Who is responsible for these acts of entextualization? Who decides whose bodies are made into what kinds of texts? And who is able to use these texts to take action? An HIV positive tattoo is very different when an HIV positive man inscribes it on himself and when a sweater company inscribes it on the body of an attractive model. Underpinning these questions, of course, are more fundamental questions of authorship, agency, and 'the political economy of texts' (Bauman and Briggs, 1990, p. 76).

Finally, these examples highlight how textual bodies influence multiple scales of human action. Such texts are not just ways of making sense of particular bodies in particular places and times. They are also means for organizing communities and institutions such as the sexual communities of barebackers, and hospitals like that in which Baldetta worked. More broadly, textual bodies are a means of organizing 'discourses'. As Berg and Bowker (1997, p. 515) put it, textual bodies and the practices of reading and writing them are implicated in the production of different people's bodies, different 'bodies politic', and different 'bodies of knowledge'.

In this chapter and the next I will consider three ways in which the body is made 'legible'. The first I call *inscription*, the act of writing upon (or 'reading off of') the surface of the body certain signs that label it as being of a certain 'type'. Inscription can be physical, as when an HIV positive person has a tattoo stating that fact inscribed onto his or her forearm, or figurative, as when a physician 'labels' a patient with a certain diagnosis. The second I call *narrativization*, the act of representing or accounting for the body in the form of a narrative. The third, which I will focus on in the next chapter, is what I call *virtualization* (Jones, 2009a, 2011; Lévy, 1998), the act of creating external representations of the body that can be separated from the physical body in time and space, recontextualized, abstracted, and combined with other texts. Here I have in mind texts such as X-rays, scans, and the results of various kinds of laboratory tests.

Of course in much of our communication about health and risk all three of these types of entextualization are present. When a patient seeks medical attention, for example, he or she normally presents the doctor with a *narrative* of what has happened to his or her body. Following from this narrative, the doctor will often create *virtual* bodies such as X-rays and test results, which will be used to perform an *inscription* – a diagnosis – onto the original body of the patient. In fact, for all of us, multiple versions of our bodies produced over the course of our lives constitute a network which implicates us in various social practices, and gives to our 'actual' bodies a specific ontology (Berg and Bowker, 1997). *Inscriptions, narratives*, and *virtual bodies* should not be seen so much as different 'kinds' of texts as different discourse practices we and others use to make our bodies into mediational means with which we perform social practices.

Inscription

By inscription I mean any process by which the body is made legible through physically or metaphorically affixing a 'label' to it. The inscription of the words 'HIV positive' onto the forearm of John Baldetta is an obvious example, and although for many this might seem a rather unusual thing to do, such inscriptions have become a common part of the way people communicate about health and risk. Scholars like Giddens (1991), Shilling (1993), and Turner (1984) have noted how self-inscription – through such acts as tattooing, tanning, working out, and cosmetic surgery – has become a feature of the hyper-reflexivity of modern life, which compels people to constantly recreate and legitimate their identities. Health has become to a large degree a matter of 'social portraiture' (Goffman, 1987), a matter of 'displaying' health for others to scrutinize (Jones, 2012). Our bodies are increasingly called upon to function as evidence of our ability to 'responsibly' monitor our own behavior when it comes to health and risk. As Finkelstein (2007) puts it, bodies have become like 'scripts' which 'tell a story about the person they embody', and learning how to make sense of such 'scripts' according to the interpretative repertories of our social groups, to 'read' health and risk off of other people's bodies, and to successfully 'write' them on our own bodies, has become a major form of 'health literacy', one which plays a much more central role in our day-to-day lives than do 'literacy practices' like reading medicine bottles and nutritional labels.

Inscriptions of health and disease are always 'written' and 'read' as part of larger systems of meaning and value. Often these outward signs of health or illness are read by others as evidence not just of our health, but also of our character, our class, or our place in society. Bourdieu (1984) has pointed out that the management of the body is central to the acquisition of status and to the maintenance of social distinctions. 'Body projects' (Featherstone, 1991) involving, for example, expensive corrective dentistry, cosmetic surgery, and tanning salons, mark the individual not just as enjoying 'health', but also as belonging to a social class which has access to such 'technologies of entextualization' (Jones, 2009a), whereas apparent 'loss of control' of one's bodily appearance, manifested in outward signs like obesity, is often associated with lower socio-economic status. At the same time, some forms of bodywork like tattoos, body piercing, and scarification can also signal subcultural identity and constitute a form of resistance to conventional notions of health and risk, as with the biohazard tattoos I discussed above (Poland and Holmes, 2009).

Issues around what bodily inscriptions mean and who has control over those meanings are central not just to the example of HIV positive tattoos I gave above, but to all forms of bodily inscription. It is an issue that is at the very heart of health and risk communication, for, as Foucault (1976, 1978–88) has famously pointed out, those who control the way meanings are made with bodies ultimately control what people are able to do with their bodies. In modern societies such control is concentrated among various 'body experts', including health professionals, counselors, personal trainers, government agencies, and pharmaceutical companies who, in the words of Shilling (1993, p. 145), 'are all involved in educating bodies and labeling as legitimate or deviant particular ways of managing and experiencing our bodies'. The body is a political surface upon which the social values and moral standards of particular communities are communicated and policed through inscriptions of 'health', 'disease', 'deviance', and 'risk' (Fox, 1993).

Diagnosis

The most important inscriptions in cases like that of John Baldetta and the 'barebackers' who inscribe biohazard tattoos onto their bodies, however, are not the tattoos they wear, but the *diagnoses* that preceded those tattoos. When it comes to health and risk, in fact, diagnosis is by far the most important kind of inscription. The writing of 'diseases' upon the body is the foundation of what Foucault (1976) called 'the medical gaze', the mechanism through which medicine claims to 'see' diseases within or upon the body. The way diagnosis is constructed in the discourse of medicine is as an act of 'reading' or deciphering the body. The 'medical gaze' is more properly thought of, however, as an act of *writing*, an act which brings diseases into being by making certain aspects of the patient's body *criterial*.

Much of the recent scholarly work on diagnosis has, building on Foucault's observations, focused on it as an exercise of power. What is emphasized is the 'cultural authority' (Starr, 1982) of doctors to 'confer' diagnoses upon patients in the same way police officers are certified to make arrests and judges are certified to deliver sentences. Research into how diagnoses are actually 'authored', however, reveals a much more complicated picture, one in which patients play an important role in co-constructing their own diagnoses. In fact, the process of diagnosis begins not with the doctor, but with the patient's decision to seek a diagnosis (Halkowski, 2006). People seek diagnoses for a variety of reasons beyond simply wishing to be 'cured' of what ails them. They also seek a way to *talk* to others about what is wrong with them, a sense that they are living in an orderly world in which conditions have 'names', and a confirmation of the legitimacy of their own bodily experiences (Hilbert, 1984).

Where applied linguistics has perhaps made its most significant contribution to the study of diagnosis is in describing how doctors and patients *work together* to *accomplish* diagnoses and make themselves mutually accountable for them (Garfinkel, 1967; Maynard, 1991; Peräkylä, 1998). Rather than simply being 'conferred' by doctors, diagnoses are contingent upon the alignment achieved between doctor and patient. The delivery of a diagnosis is often 'fraught with interactional tensions' (Maynard, 2004; see also Peräkylä, 1998) in which the authority of the doctor must be reconciled with the patient's intimate knowledge of his or her own body. In order to achieve this alignment, doctors often frame diagnoses as 'joint activities'. The following example from Maynard (2004) illustrates how doctors sometimes invite patients to take part in formulating diagnoses.

01	Dr H:	Do you remember we said we saw something g:ro:wing in your
02		stomach? =
03	Mr J:	-Mm hm
04		(0.6)
05	Dr H:	D' you remember that?
06		(0.6)
07	Mr J:	Ye:ah I guess.
08	Dr H:	= oh kay. Well that's what we did see:. We looked into your
09		stomach and we sa:w: (0.6) right at the spo:t where you
10		feel like (0.2) the food is getting stu:ck,
11		(0.1)
12	Mr J:	Mm
13		(1.0)
14	Dr H:	M.hhh uh:, there is something growing in your stomach.
15		(4.0)
16	Mr J:	You can't tell what it is? =
17	Dr H:	I can tell you what it is Clint.
18		(0.1)
19	Mr J:	Mm hm.
20		(0.1)
21	Dr H:	Uh: (0.2) it's cancer.

22   (0.4)
23   Mr J: Jhheesuhhs: *(Maynard, 2004, p. 69)*

Although the patient in this example cannot be said to contribute much to the diagnostic reasoning, the doctor is extremely careful to construe the act of examining the evidence as a kind of 'joint seeing' ('Do you remember *we* said *we* saw something … '). More important, however, is how the doctor avoids actually diagnosing the patient, focusing instead on characterizing the evidence ('*it's* cancer.'). This might seem like a subtle distinction, but, as Maynard argues, this slight distancing of the diagnosis from the patient allows the doctor the opportunity to assess how easy it will be for the patient to accept the diagnosis. As Maynard puts it, 'clinicians may cite evidence not just because of an interest in sharing laboratory or other findings with patients or family members but as an inexplicit way to predicate a disease as an attribute of the person' (p. 70). At the end of this encounter it is the *patient*, not the doctor, who finally ends up explicitly diagnosing himself, while the doctor continues to hedge: after the doctor suggests that he will feel better after surgery, the patient replies:

Mr J: But I still got cancer. (0.5)
Dr H: That ma:y be the case. (70)

This linguistic negotiation regarding where to *locate* the diagnosis is something that the patient carries out of the examining room and into his or her subsequent encounters with friends, family members employers, insurers, and other healthcare workers. How does he or she explain to others what has happened? Staiano (1986) draws an important distinction between what it means to say 'I am' (for example, a diabetic), and 'I have' or 'I suffer from' a disease like diabetes. The first (existential) construction posits the disease as defining the self, the second (possessive) construes it as something external that the individual possesses, and the third construes it as an experience that the individual is undergoing. Fleischman (1999) uses her own experience of being diagnosed with *myelodysplasia* as an example of how people use such constructions strategically to either identify with or distance themselves from their diagnoses. She writes:

> For a period of time after being diagnosed I would respond to the question, 'What do you have?' by saying, '*I've been diagnosed with myelodysplasia.*' This construction involves a verb in the passive-voice and one that licenses the interpretation that I may not in fact have the disease at all, I've just been diagnosed with it. But as time went on, and I came to accept the fact of living (perhaps permanently) with MDS, I found myself migrating toward the 'I have' construction, though the object of that verb would – and still does – vary, depending on the level of biological knowledge I attribute to my addressee or the emotional wallop I wish my utterance to pack. Though nothing changes in my body depending on whether I say I have a refractory

anemia or I have a rare disorder of the bone-marrow or I have a fatal blood disease – all accurate characterizations of my situation – what I communicate by means of these respective referring expressions is quite different.

(p. 9)

Diagnosis – as with so many other acts of naming – is a matter not just of describing the world, but of taking strategic action in it. The 'value' of a diagnosis to a doctor or a patient often has less to do with how 'true' it is, as with its utility as a text which the patient (or the physician) can subsequently appropriate to take other actions, like making an insurance claim. While most people focus on the way diagnoses *limit* social action, it is important to remember that diagnoses also serve as entitlements: they allow patients to obtain funds for medical treatment, claim the right to be absent from work, receive social benefits, and in some cases (such as murder trials) escape punishment for crimes they have committed. Doctors, of course, are well aware of the pragmatic utility of their diagnoses, and sometimes make them based more on the kinds of entitlements they think patients should receive than on an objective assessment of their condition. In his book *Unstrange Minds* (2007, p. 130), for example, anthropologist Roy Richard Grinker points out that many clinicians evaluating children for autism 'are more likely to give a child a diagnosis that he or she thinks will help the child receive the best services or school placement than a diagnosis that conforms to the *Diagnostic and Statistical Manual*.' Patients are also increasingly aware of the kinds of entitlements certain diagnoses bring and often not shy about approaching physicians in order to obtain them. Pediatric psychologist Lawrence Diller (2006), for instance, reveals how some parents bring their teenage children to be evaluated for attention deficit hyperactivity disorder (ADHD) soon before the children are scheduled to sit for public examinations, knowing that such a diagnosis will bring with it not only drugs that they believe will help their children study, but also the possibility of a special dispensation allowing them to spend more time taking the test.

Most pragmatic uses of diagnoses in everyday life, however, are not so cynical. They involve patients or their carers making moment-by-moment strategic decisions about whether or not to deploy certain diagnoses in order to solve immediate problems. Mary Foster-Galasso (2005) provides an excellent illustration of this in her description of how she and her husband cope with her son's diagnosis with 'pervasive developmental disorder, not otherwise specified' (PDD-NOS), a label which is difficult to explain to most people. She relates, for example, an incident which occurred between her son and a fellow parishioner in her church:

> My son Calvin ... is eleven. Back when he was about seven, we were shaking hands and saying, 'Peace be with you' at a key point in the Catholic Mass, when Calvin suddenly shattered our family's peace by asking the older woman beside him – in his too-high-pitched, just slightly off 'normal' voice, and of course standing just a tad too close, so he could practically look up her nostrils – 'Why do you have that big moustache?'

I tried to hush him and look apologetic, but neither my husband Gary nor I could say more, because the congregation is totally silent in the next part of the Mass. By the end of the service, I thought the incident was all over. But it wasn't. As soon as the final notes of the recessional hymn died away, she was waiting for us, blocking our path to the aisle, her large body a mass of indignation, displaying her wounded feelings, and just waiting to give us a piece of her mind. 'I've been watching you at church. You can't control that little rascal.'

I tried to make excuses. 'I'm sorry about what Calvin said. He has a problem with what to say, because he's got a type of autism' ... I'd used a diagnosis word, offering it up like an appeasement, or perhaps a hope for some shared understanding. Understand us better, maybe even pity us if you want, but step aside and let us get into the aisle and out of here. Now.

The diagnosis word had its effect; one I hadn't intended: 'Well, you know, there are places for people like him.'

(pp. 17–18)

This story provides a dramatic example of how diagnoses function (or fail to function) in people's attempts to make themselves accountable for themselves and those for whom they are caring. Here Foster-Galasso uses a label she believes is most likely to 'excuse' her son for his inappropriate behavior and elicit sympathy from the woman. Unfortunately, it has the opposite effect, further stigmatizing him. What Foster-Galasso's experiences highlight is the degree to which diagnoses are highly contingent and unstable, even *after* they have been delivered by physicians.

The process of diagnosis, like the 'body projects' I discussed above, always takes place within larger institutional and social regimes and is often governed by economic and political forces that extend beyond the consultation room. While they function to constrain and amplify the social actions of individual doctors and patients, diagnoses also function to constrain and amplify the actions of institutions like hospitals, schools, insurance companies, and pharmaceutical companies, facilitating things like surveillance, administration, marketing, and billing, and what diagnoses can be given and what they can subsequently be used for often involves a complex process of negotiation among these institutions. There has been considerable research, for example, on how the definition of conditions like post-traumatic stress disorder (PTSD) (Armstrong, 1995), fibromyalgia (Stabile, 1992), and adult attention deficit/hyperactivity disorder (Conrad, 2007) are shaped by political and economic forces, as well as on the role of the pharmaceutical industry in creating and 'branding' new diseases (Moynihan and Cassels, 2005; Parry, 2003; Payer, 1992).

These institutional forces can have a direct and dramatic impact on how diagnoses are actually authored in clinical settings. Diller (2006) notes how the administrative requirements of insurance companies have come more and more to shape interactions between doctors and patients. Reimbursement protocols are structured so as to reward doctors for short visits that result in a clear diagnosis and a prescription. It has become much more difficult for doctors to refrain from giving a diagnosis, to express uncertainty, or to limit treatment to 'non-billable' measures like suggestions that patients alter their behavior.

The main point I'm trying to make is that diagnosis is not simply a matter of a doctor 'inscribing' a condition onto the body of a patient. It is a complex social practice that involves doctors, institutions like schools, scientific committees, and insurance companies and drug companies. A diagnosis can function as a means for performing a whole host of different kinds of social actions for all of the different 'stakeholders' involved. At the same time, it also functions as a kind of 'glue' that helps to sustain the complex web of relationships among these different participants.

Narrativization

Whereas diagnosis is a way of entextualizing the body based on the interpretation of signs and symptoms, narrativization is a way of presenting the body as a *consequence* of actions and experiences (Schiffrin, 1996). In the last chapter I looked at ways of analyzing narratives in order to understand how people organize and account for risk behavior. Here I am more concerned with narratives of illness as means by which people perform social practices and claim and impute social identities.

Like diagnosis, narrative is a form of discourse with a long history in medicine. Before the popularization of biomedical models of disease in the nineteenth century, in fact, patients' narratives were the primary texts through which doctors came to know the bodies of their patients. Bury (2001) describes how in the seventeenth and eighteenth centuries, doctors were unlikely to perform physical examinations of their patients at all, but rather based their diagnoses and treatment recommendations entirely on patients' narratives, which involved information not just about the patient's physical condition, but also about his or her lifestyle, relationships, and the wider environment in which he or she lived.

Although the importance of narrative as a diagnostic tool has decreased considerably over the years, especially with the development of new technologies of entextualization which enable physicians to 'look inside' the bodies of their patients (Armstrong, 1984; see chapter 7), many have argued that the 'logic' of narrative pervades many of the most basic social practices in medicine from clinical rounds and case reports (Good, 1994; Hunter, 1993) to notations on medical charts (Poirier and Brauner, 1990). Some have even gone so far as to suggest that medical knowledge itself has an essentially narrative structure (Brody, 1987; Greenhalgh, 1998). At the same time, as I mentioned in chapter 3, narrative has also been seen as a form of entextualization which is in some ways *at odds with* the analytical modes of thinking that dominate modern medical practices (Bruner, 1985). As Mishler (1984) has famously pointed out, sometimes patients' stories are regarded by doctors as distracting from rather than contributing to the business of diagnosis. Different processes of entextualization, as I have been emphasizing throughout this book, operate to make different aspects of our experience criterial and to construct things (like 'diseases' and 'health') and people (like 'patients' and 'doctors') differently. Diagnostic practices that rely on analytical, 'evidence-based' models operate to decontextualize the patient's experiences and generalize about them based on their similarity to particular 'classes' of experiences identified in wider populations. Narrativization, on the other hand, operates to particularize the patient's experiences and place them in a specific temporal and social context (Polkinghorne, 1988).

Partly as a result of the insights of researchers like Mishler, since the 1980s there has been an increased interest in the therapeutic and diagnostic value of patient narratives, what Polkinghorne (1988) refers to as a 'narrative turn' in the field of medicine. The literature on illness narrative that has accumulated in the past three decades is vast and varied, focusing on such aspects of narrative as how it is used by patients to 'make sense' of their illness experiences (see, for example, Clarke et al., 2003; Kleinman, 1988; Ochberg, 1988), how illness narratives appropriate larger cultural storylines (see, for example, Frank, 1995), how patients and doctors co-construct narratives (see, for example, Clark and Mishler, 1992), and the role of illness narratives in the construction of social identities (see, for example, Riessman, 1990). More recently there has been a strong movement to restore narrative to a central place in clinical practice. Known as 'narrative-based medicine', a term chosen deliberately to contrast it with 'evidence-based medicine' (Greenhalgh, 1998), this movement advocates a more holistic approach to patients, which focuses not just on their physical symptoms but also on the way these symptoms are contextualized through the stories they tell. Narratives are promoted for their utility both in helping patients to come to terms with their illness and in helping doctors formulate more accurate diagnoses and more appropriate treatments (Charon, 2001; Elwyn and Gwyn, 1999; Greenhalgh and Hurwitz, 1998).

There are, however, those who have expressed reservations about the enthusiasm with which narrative has been embraced as a research tool in the study of health and illness. Paul Atkinson and David Silverman (Atkinson, 1997, 2009; Atkinson and Silverman, 1997), for example, point out that for many social scientists, patients' narratives have come to be regarded as unproblematic representations of actual experiences or unproblematic reflections of patients' states of mind. This 'naïve realism', they argue, is often coupled with a kind of 'romanticism' which privileges the narratives of patients as 'true' and 'authentic' while denigrating the analytical reasoning of biomedicine as 'artificial' and 'sterile'.

The most important criticism Atkinson and Silverman level at narrative-based approaches to the study of health and illness is that in most cases narratives are treated as 'free-floating', decontextualized entities rather than as socially occasioned instances of discourse. Indeed, in most studies of illness narratives, the narratives analyzed are elicited in the context of research interviews, which bear little resemblance to the real-life situations in which narratives naturally occur. This does not necessarily make them less valid as data. The problem is not so much that they are not 'naturally occurring', but that they are analyzed with little or no reference to the social situation of their production.

Although most applied linguists are not as skeptical of narrative approaches to the study of health and illness, they do share with Atkinson and Silverman the conviction that the analysis of narrative must begin with a consideration of its *social* dimensions. Like all texts, narratives are a matter of social action, and so must be approached with an eye not just to what they 'mean', but also what they *do* in the particular social situations in which they are produced and consumed. Individuals who produce narratives do not speak 'alone, about themselves and for themselves, in a social vacuum' (Atkinson, 2009, para. 2.14), but rather as socially situated speakers speaking to socially situated listeners in specific social situations for specific reasons.

There are three main features of an applied linguistic approach to narrative analysis that distinguish it from the approaches taken by other social sciences. First, applied linguists consider 'the "how" of the telling ... as important as the "what" that is said' (Riessman, 1990, p. 1196). They are particularly concerned with the ways storytellers use tools of entextualization like those I discussed in chapter 3 to construct certain 'versions' of events and certain 'versions' of people. Second, applied linguists are concerned with stories as *purposive* and *occasioned* pieces of discourse, mindful of the relationship of a story's content and form to the concrete social actions the story is used to take. Third, they see stories as both *dialogic* and *heteroglossic*, always co-constructed by storytellers and their audiences and involving the mixing of multiple 'voices'.

Story and structure

As part of his critique of the way many social scientists approach narrative, Atkinson (2009) makes the rather bold statement that, for narrative analysis to really constitute a valid analytical project, 'the analysis of form should take precedence over the thematic analysis of content' (para. 3.9). What he means by this is not that content is unimportant, but that what people say in their narratives cannot be properly interpreted without taking into account the processes of entextualization they have used to make certain aspects of their experience criterial and to imbue their actions with logic and significance.

The resources narrators use to structure their discourse include the kinds of words they use and the broader systems of classification invoked by those choices, the ways they combine grammatical participants and processes together to construct actions and events and to assign agency, and the ways they use things like pronouns, evaluative words, and the language's systems of modality and modulation to construct relationships with their audience. Where analysts of narrative from an applied linguistic perspective often begin in their analysis, however, is with the overall organization of the narrative.

The classic approach to narrative organization in applied linguistics comes from the work of Labov and Waletzsky (1967), who developed their framework by isolating the recurrent features in a large corpus of narratives gathered from sociolinguistic interviews. Narratives, they found, tend to consist of a number of distinctive phases which they call (1) the abstract (a short summarizing statement that signals that a story is about to begin; (2) the orientation (a description of the setting, the time of the events, and the people involved); (3) the complication (one or more incidents that are problematic and so make the story worth telling); (4) the resolution (a description of how the complication/s was/were resolved); (5) the evaluation (a commentary on the events which serves to make the point of the story clear); and (6) the coda (which signals that the story has ended and brings the listener back into the present moment). Of course many narratives do not conform exactly to this pattern. Often, for example, the abstract or coda is left off, or the evaluation is embedded within the other sections rather than constituting a section of its own. The kind of information given in the orientation and the number and ordering of complications can also vary a great deal from narrative to narrative. In a way, the real value of this heuristic is not to help us to see structural similarities across different narratives, but to give us a way to notice the *variations* across narratives and to understand how storytellers use these variations to frame their stories in particular ways or to highlight some aspects of what happened and background other aspects.

Consider the following simple narrative told by a 23-year-old HIV positive British man in Hong Kong in the context of a focus group with other HIV positive patients in which they were asked to discuss factors influencing the quality of life of people with HIV/AIDS.

```
01   A:  Yes ... well when I first got it, I played rugby ... a pretty intense form, and
02       then I got this diagnosis and it was fine for a while, but then the CD4
03       started to drop down and so I decided to take it (antiretroviral
04       treatment) earlier ... I mean, I really just wanted to attack it as quickly
05       as possible.
```

Although this story is extremely short, it contains nearly all of the elements in Labov and Waletzsky's model. The storyteller begins by signaling that he is about to tell a story with the words, 'Yes ... well', and then goes on to orient the listener to the topic and timeframe of the story (when he was first diagnosed with HIV) and the relevant circumstances of that time frame (the fact that he was playing rugby). He then proceeds with a series of complicating clauses describing getting the diagnosis, being fine for 'a while', and then seeing his CD4 count drop down, and a resolution, deciding to begin antiretroviral treatment. It ends with an evaluation which explains not just why he decided to begin treatment but gives thematic coherence to the whole story as an illustration of the teller's approach to dealing with his infection – 'attacking' it. This is not so much a story about getting HIV as it is about 'fighting' HIV, and framed in this way, the reference to rugby at the beginning does not just index the teller's pre-infection life of health and normality, but also plays into the central metaphor of the story – that of dealing with HIV as a kind of contest or battle.

Sometimes when people tell stories in conversations they tell them more than once, elaborating or reframing their accounts in their retellings. That is exactly what happens in this instance. In response to another participant in the focus group asking for clarification regarding a detail in his story (his CD4 count), the storyteller reformulates the same story, further developing the theme that he introduced in the first telling.

06 B: What was the count?
07 A: The count … well, when I was first diagnosed, the count was actually
08   quite high. 590. VL 19,000. Now this is very interesting 'cause once
09   you know you are mentally stressed, I mean you go negative, and you
10   can actually get worse very quickly. You might have this thing for six
11   years, and you don't even know you've got it, so you don't have to cope
12   mentally. Your body is responding and staying fit. But when you know,
13   you start thinking of yourself as sick. So believe it or not, when I went
14   for another blood test, the CD4 for no apparent reason had gone down
15   to 480. 'Cause I was worrying myself sick … a hundred points … I'm
16   talking about two months later. And the VL shot up to 130,000 … no
17   apparent reason, just mental degeneration. So you've got to pick
18   yourself back up and keep going. The whole thing is now back up to
19   somewhere around 700 to 800 and VL down to nothing. And basically
20   I'm trying to play rugby again, but the drugs have an effect on my
        joints.

Whereas in the first telling of the story, rugby playing is thematized (as a metaphor for the teller's pre-infection life), in this retelling it serves more of an evaluative function, illustrating the effectiveness of the narrator's change in attitude and the transformation of his health condition. One particularly striking aspect of this story is the construction of the laboratory tests as the active agents in it. The teller's CD4 count 'goes down' and his viral load 'shoots up' seemingly of their own volition ('for no apparent reason'). In contrast to the active portrayal of the laboratory tests, the speaker portrays himself as mostly passive, engaged in mental processes ('knowing', 'thinking', 'believing', 'worrying', and 'going negative'). Even when his health is good (before the diagnosis is actually revealed to him), it is not him, but his 'body' that is 'responding and staying fit'. The turning point of the story comes when the teller escapes from the downward spiral of obsessive mental processes and reclaims the ability to act upon the material world by doing something ('trying to play rugby'). It is important to note that this change of attitude is construed not as a mental process, but as a material one ('picking oneself up').

Another striking thing about this narrative is the teller's use of pronouns. In almost the entire story, except for the very beginning and the very end, he uses the second person pronoun ('you') to represent himself, rather than the first person. The primary effect of this is to generalize his experiences, to present them as things that have (or might have) happened to his audience as well as himself. This generalization is further accomplished by the shift to the present tense, transforming what began as a situated narrative to what Riessman (1990) calls a 'habitual narrative'. With this technique the narrator is able to give to his personal experiences a universal significance so that his evaluation of what happened to him also functions as advice for his listeners ('You've got to pick yourself back up').

Cheshire and Ziebland (2005) note that 'habitual narratives' are especially associated with patients with chronic illnesses, since chronic illness inevitably involves the reoccurrence of symptoms and the routinization of actions to manage those symptoms. At the same time it might be argued that there is something inherently dangerous about this mode of storytelling in the context of chronic disease since it can reify the experience of the disease and limit opportunities for transformative thinking (Frank, 1995). What is interesting in the example above is how the speaker uses a habitual narrative as a *means* of illustrating the dangers inherent in habitual thinking.

What we do with stories

When people tell stories they do so in order to accomplish one or more social actions. The narrator above tells his story not just to communicate his experience, but also to create solidarity with the other people in the group and to give them advice. This is what we mean when we say that stories are *purposive* and *occasioned*. No matter what the circumstances, people tell stories in order to *do* things, and the form and content of stories cannot really be properly understood without reference to their social functions. Such functions might include eliciting sympathy, building solidarity, gaining access to some goods or services, claiming exemption from some obligation, or justifying a particular state of affairs.

Often these social functions occur in the context of professional or institutional encounters in which narratives contribute to clear, instrumental goals. Such an institutional setting might be, for example, a clinical situation in which a patient narrates the story of his or her symptoms to a doctor or therapist in order to provide the doctor with evidence with which to make a diagnosis. Most doctors begin consultations by eliciting patient narratives and, at least in the beginning, usually surrender the floor to the patient for a longer period than at any other time in the consultation (Pomerantz et al., 2007; Stivers and Heritage, 2001). Chatwin (2006) explores ways in which doctors use various strategies to aid patients in constructing narratives by, for example, not interrupting, showing interest, and refraining from introducing new topics before patients' accounts are allowed to come to their 'natural end'. At the same time, he notes, patients are often cooperative in making sure that what they choose to include in their narratives is relevant. In other words, patients routinely 'self-censor' their narratives, trying to produce stories which they believe their doctors will find 'useful'.

Nevertheless, as I have mentioned before, there is substantial evidence that doctors frequently interrupt patient narratives, take them in another direction, or attempt to control them through questions in ways which cause the stories to lose their narrative coherence and become fragmented (see, for example, Clark and Mishler, 1992; Slade et al., 2008). The main reason for this is that doctors and patients often regard the functions of narratives in rather different ways. The evidentiary function of the narrative, which is so central to the doctor's interpretative framework, may be, for the patient, only one of many reasons for telling their story. Patients may also be using the story to seek confirmation of their experiences, to show that they are a particular kind of patient, to complain about someone (a family member, another doctor), or even to gain access to a *particular* diagnosis or a particular drug.

Scholars of narrative-based medicine point out that sometimes patients see narratives not as an aid to diagnosis, but rather as a *counter-text* to it, an attempt to resist 'the transformation of the person one always thought one was into a "patient with a diagnosis"' (Greenhalgh, 2001, p. 324). 'Crafting our personal narratives,' says Greenhalgh, 'is a way to keep our lives our own, to protect all or part of our identities from threat or assault' (p. 342). Young (1989) provides a particularly poignant example of this in his description of a physical examination of an elderly Jewish university professor during which the professor resists the medicalization of the self by recounting, as the doctor moves from one bodily part to another, his experiences as an inmate of Auschwitz. These stories, argues Young, help the patient maintain a sense of his social and 'historical' self in the face of the decontextualizing logic of diagnosis.

There is much less research on how people use illness narratives to get things done in non-institutional settings, in their daily lives at work or with their families (but see, for example, Beach, 2001; van Dijck, 2005). Often, of course, accounts of the body in such situations differ dramatically from those given in doctors' offices since, in most cultural contexts, outside of institutional encounters the sick are often encouraged to downplay rather than highlight their condition so as to avoid creating embarrassment for themselves and for the healthy people around them. It is by being sick but acting well that people show themselves as worthy of the care and sympathy of others (Radley and Billig, 1996). Nevertheless, illness narratives can sometimes be deployed as a way of justifying behavior that might otherwise be regarded as unacceptable or inappropriate. Riessman (1990), for example, shows how people in the process of divorce seek to excuse their behavior by blaming it on illness. People also regularly tell stories for or about people they are caring for, as, for example, when parents give accounts of children with handicaps (Voysey, 2006) or the carers of elderly people suffering from dementia or Alzheimer's take part in helping the people they are caring for initiate and complete narratives (Crichton and Koch, 2011). As with everyday narratives told by ill people themselves, the purpose of narratives told about others is often to enact 'normality' rather than to call attention to a disease or medical condition.

One reason there are so few examples of everyday illness narratives in the literature is due to the very *occasioned* nature of such narratives, and the difficulty for analysts to predict and prepare for the many kinds of social occasions which might give rise to them. As a consequence, we are often forced to settle for narratives that are occasioned by more 'artificial' activities such as research interviews. As I said above, this in itself is not bad, as long as we take into account the ways such occasions are regarded by participants and what they use them to try to accomplish. The focus groups we conducted on the quality of life of people living with HIV, for example, were often used by participants as opportunities to exchange advice and give and receive mutual support, as can be seen in the exchange analyzed above involving the HIV-positive rugby player. They were also often used as occasions to complain about hospital services since participants believed that researchers might have influence with doctors or others in positions of power.

'Voices' in narrative

As should already be clear from the discussion above, narratives cannot be considered the sole property of those who produce them. They presuppose an audience, and both the identity of the audience and their reaction to the unfolding narrative have an effect on the eventual shape the narrative takes. Audience members are basically 'co-authors' (Duranti, 1986) who contribute to the story by making certain kinds of demands upon the teller and giving evidence of how they judge the story. The most obvious example of this is in medical encounters in which patients construct their narratives in relation to the questions that their doctors ask (Cicourel, 1983; Eggly, 2002). Another example is how participants in both formal and informal group discussions cooperate in helping one another construct their stories, offering evaluative comments, asking clarification questions, and taking up themes or problems from previous tellers and incorporating them into their own narratives. In fact, one of the chief advantages of using focus groups as a research methodology is that they give analysts a chance to witness the social dynamics of such dialogism (Hydén and Bülow, 2003).

Much of the therapeutic benefit of narrativization appears to be associated with its dialogic character. While the contributions of doctors and therapists in asymmetrical professional encounters have often been seen as compromising patients' ability to tell their stories, they can also serve to encourage patients to elaborate or help them to focus their narratives (Chatwin, 2006). It is particularly in discussions between patients, however, in contexts like 'support groups' (Humphreys, 2000; Jensen, 2000), online forums and blogs (Hamilton, 1998; Page, 2012), and even focus group interviews designed to elicit data (Hydén and Bülow, 2003; Lehoux et al., 2006), that the therapeutic potential of narratives has been most frequently observed. Co-narrativization is an important means through which people make sense of their experiences by getting other people's reactions to them, cultivate a feeling that they 'are not alone', and work together with others to solve problems (Ochs et al., 1989).

Bülow (2004), in her analysis of discussions among sufferers of chronic fatigue syndrome, noted three distinct patterns of dialogism in group storytelling. The first, which she refers to as the *self-contained personal narrative*, consists of individuals relating their personal experiences to a group, much like the example I analyzed above of the HIV-positive rugby player. What makes such narratives dialogic is not just the fact that the verbal and non-verbal reactions of the audience help to shape the way narrators tell their stories, but that narrators themselves necessarily construct stories in ways which suit their audiences and 'fit' into interactions (Sacks, 1995). In the narrative analyzed above, for instance, the speaker's story is constructed not just to meet his own needs of self-expression, but also to address the needs of his listeners whom he believes are suffering similar problems.

The second form of co-narrativization noted by Bülow is what she calls *orchestrated chained personal stories*. These consist of a series of stories told in some kind of organized fashion, often facilitated by a moderator. The stories that recovering alcoholics tell at AA meetings fall into this category. What makes these stories dialogic is not just the reactions and cooperative interruptions from listeners, but also the way people build on and reflect one another's stories structurally and thematically. When AA members take turns telling their stories, they are all producing individualized versions of what they regard as their 'common story'. Listening to and telling stories in a chained manner has the power to facilitate the 'reflective self-awareness' that is necessary for generative explorations of the self (O'Reilly, 1997).

The third way participants in Bülow's study co-constructed their narratives, and the most frequent format she observed, is what she calls *co-narrated collectivized stories*. These occur when participants spontaneously engage in 'constructing a joint story using several participants' experiences or by evaluating and elaborating another participant's personal experiences' (Bülow, 2004, p. 45). Often, says Bülow, each person's contribution is less than what would usually be considered a full story, but taken collectively they come to constitute a coherent narrative message.

An example of this type of co-narrativization can be seen in an exchange which occurred immediately after the story I analyzed above, which the narrator ended by problematizing his physical response to antiretroviral drugs ('I'm trying to play rugby again, but the drugs have an effect on my joints'). In what followed, two listeners (B and C) joined with the first narrator in taking up the theme of 'not giving in to anxiety or despair' by cooperatively generating a number of alternative versions of what was essentially the same story.

21	B:	I have that problem now.
22	A:	I think the joints … I got a lot of problems going on in my legs cause
23		I play rugby … I can still play but I can't run as much anymore, I can't
24		make the distance …
25	B:	You feel it here (rubbing his knees).
26	C:	I got the same thing. You know, I trained in the service 10 years ago.
27		And now I find when I try to lift weights I feel old … you know I can feel
28		my joints and feel it in the back and my thighs and everything. Even
29		your hands and fingers … I've had a pain in my thumb for a couple of
30		weeks and I don't understand why …
31	A:	But I think you can't obsess about …
32	B:	The point is if that happened to you and you didn't know you're
33		positive, I think it wouldn't freak you out so much …
34	A:	You wouldn't immediately think, 'Oh my god! I am gonna be a
35		cripple' …
36	B:	I was on holiday and started coughing, and all I could think was,
37		'Oh my God! Maybe it's PCP'
38	C:	You can drive yourself crazy.

39   A: You get tired and you think 'it's because of my HIV', but then you look
40   at all the people around you at work, and they're all tired too. So you
41   gotta be careful.

In the beginning of this exchange, B and C take up the complication that arose from A's previous narrative about the importance of avoiding negative thinking. As they do, however, they actually begin to engage in just the kind of negative thinking A warns against, producing anecdotes of their physical difficulties, until A returns to his original theme ('But I think you can't obsess … '). At this point, both B and C join him in producing a series of short narratives to illustrate this point. Again we can see the use of 'habitual narrative', with both A and B using the pronoun 'you' in lines 31–35, and A again using it at the very end of the excerpt. Whereas in A's narrative, analyzed above, A's use of habitual narrative served to set up a contrast between what 'normally' happens to people when they are diagnosed and how he in particular broke out of those habitual patterns, here it seems to function more to facilitate the transformation of personal experience into a shared collectivized experience. As the collectivized story progresses, participants alternate between particularized versions (using 'I') and generalized versions (using 'you') (see Figure 6.2). Each time an individual experience is introduced, participants work together to turn it into something that they all understand and share.

Through these exercises in co-narrativization, says Bülow (2004), people are able to create a shared understanding of their predicament. They are also able to confirm and legitimate one another's individual suffering. Most importantly, narrativization gives them a way to dialogically 'work through' their problems, coming up with joint solutions and helping one another to apply these general solutions to their particular circumstances.

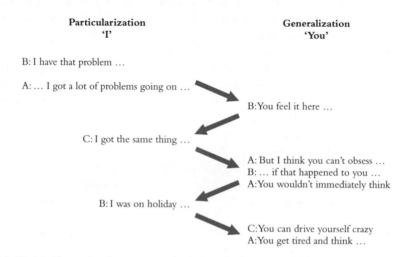

FIGURE 6.2 Alternation between particularization and generalization

Along with being dialogic, narratives are also heteroglossic. Narrators construct them through appropriating various stock phrases, stereotypical plots, recognizable characters, and other cultural conventions as well as by appropriating the words, thoughts, and actions of the other people who play a part in their stories. As I noted in chapter 2, the ways people choose to represent the voices of others (and of their own 'past selves') in narratives through direct quotation, paraphrase, or more subtly through things like presupposition, function to position tellers in relation to these different voices. One of the challenges in analyzing voice appropriation and discourse representation, however, is that it is difficult to make generalizations about the effect different forms of discourse representation have outside of the context of particular texts and their use in particular social situations. Several analysts, for example, have taken up the issue of reported speech in patients' narratives of their interactions with healthcare workers and the way it reveals underlying inequalities. Cheshire and Ziebland (2005), for example, equate, direct speech with power. The higher power patients attribute to doctors, they claim, is reflected in the fact that 'what doctors say tends to be reported in the form of direct speech whereas what the patients themselves say is more likely to be reported as indirect speech' (p. 29). Hamilton (1998), on the other hand, as I discussed in chapter 2, notes that in the stories told by the bone marrow transplant survivors whom she analyzes, narrators sometimes attribute direct speech to doctors as a way of distancing themselves from them and demonstrating their callousness to readers.

To understand the relationship between discourse representation and power, one must look at the specific circumstances in which speech is quoted, summarized, or otherwise characterized and take note of a range of accompanying features such as the verbs of reporting and other evaluative tools the narrator uses. The story below from an internet forum (Torrey, 2011) in which a woman reports her frustrations surrounding being misdiagnosed with a rare form of cancer illustrates the multiple ways reported speech can be used.

01 In late June 2004, I found a golf ball-sized lump on my torso. It didn't hurt – it
02 was just there.
03 I immediately made an appointment with my family doctor and, because he
04 had no idea what it was, he sent me to a surgeon who removed it that
05 afternoon. 'We'll let you know when we hear back from the lab,' was the
06 surgeon's departing comment as I pulled my shirt back on and got ready to
07 go home.
08 A week later, no word. I contacted the surgeon's office and was told the
09 results weren't back yet. The Fourth of July holiday had caused the delay, so I
10 waited.
11 Another week later, the surgeon finally called me with my lab results. 'You
12 have a very rare cancer called subcutaneous panniculitis-like T-cell
13 lymphoma,' he told me.
14 And then he dropped a second bomb. I was told that the reason the lab
15 results took so long was because the outcome was so rare – that a second lab

16 had been called for a second opinion. 'Two labs have independently
17 confirmed these results,' I was told. 'We'll make an oncology appointment
18 for you as soon as possible.'
19 'As soon as possible' took more than two weeks, not unusual as I'm sure you
20 know if you've ever needed an oncology appointment. I immediately began
21 searching the Internet for information about subcutaneous panniculitis-like
22 T-cell lymphoma (SPTCL). It was hard to find anything at all because, as the
23 surgeon had told me, it's very rare.
24 What I did learn was that it was a terminal, fast-acting disease. (I understand
25 a treatment protocol has more recently been developed that extends life for
26 up to two years.) The longest anyone with SPTCL seemed to live was a couple
27 of years, regardless of whether or not they received any treatment.
28 When I finally saw the oncologist, he was very discouraging. Dr. S, I'll call
29 him, sent me for blood work and a CT scan, both of which came back negative
30 for any abnormalities. Yet he insisted the lab work trumped the lack of other
31 evidence.
32 It just didn't make sense to me. I felt fine. I was playing golf once or twice a
33 week. I just knew pieces were missing.
34 When I pushed him for more information, he cited my additional symptoms
35 hot flashes and night sweats. 'But I'm 52!' I admonished. 'At 52 all women
36 have night sweats and hot flashes!'
37 He insisted my symptoms were unrelated to menopause. Instead, he said,
38 they were symptoms of my lymphoma. Without chemo, he told me, I would
39 be dead by the end of the year.
40 I asked about the possibility that the lab results were wrong. 'No – not a
41 chance', he said. Two labs had independently confirmed the results. The
42 pressure to start chemotherapy began to mount.
43 Besides my family and a few close friends, I didn't share the news with
44 anyone else. My business was already suffering – being self-employed and
45 having lousy health insurance meant that my diagnosis had now become
46 expensive, too. I was spending way too much time researching, fretting, and
47 paying for doctor visits and tests that were only marginally covered by my
48 insurance. Life, what was left of it, was going down the tubes – fast.
49 By then it was August, and I had a decision to make. Chemo, or no chemo? I
50 learned that Dr. S had taken sick, and his partner Dr. H was taking over my
51 case. Dr. H asked me why I was waiting to begin chemo, and I told him I was
52 trying to find another oncologist for a second opinion. There were too many
53 question marks. His reply to me makes me shudder to this day, 'What you
54 have is so rare, no one will know any more about it than I do.'
55 If anything compelled me to begin digging deeper, that was it. Now I was
56 'sick' AND angry!

As with the stories analyzed by Cheshire and Ziebland (2005) and Hamilton
(1998), the speech of the doctors in this narrative is represented much more

frequently as direct speech and that of the narrator is more frequently reported as indirect speech. While the direct speech of the doctors does serve to portray them as occupying positions of power, the narrator, like Hamilton's bone marrow transplant survivors, also uses discourse representation skillfully to call the legitimacy of that power into question. One way she does this is through the words she uses to report the speech of the doctors. Rather than using active verbs of reporting (for example, 'he said … ' or 'he explained … '), she often characterizes the doctors' speech either using nouns ('"We'll let you know when we hear back from the lab," was the surgeon's departing comment … '), or passive voice verbs ('"Two labs have independently confirmed these results," I was told'). This has the effect of portraying the doctors' manner of speaking as impersonal and bureaucratic. The use of direct speech by doctors also makes them vulnerable to having their words parodied or used as evidence against them, as in line 19 when the doctor's words 'As soon as possible' are repeated to demonstrate how unreliable the doctor's words were.

At the same time, the place in the story in which the patient's words are reported as direct speech and the doctor's words are reported as indirect speech (lines 35–38) does not represent a reversal of roles, with the patient becoming powerful and the doctor becoming more passive. On the contrary, the use of discourse representation in this passage works to reinforce the frustration the narrator feels in dealing with unresponsive doctors. Her own use of direct speech to challenge the doctor ('"But I'm 52!" I admonished. "At 52 all women have night sweats and hot flashes!"') is met not with reciprocal direct speech, but rather with indirectly reported acts of 'citing' (line 35) and 'insisting' (line 38) which make the doctor's reaction to the narrator's seemingly reasonable concerns seem cursory and dismissive. Here indirect speech is used to highlight the doctor's words as constituting what Bakhtin (1986) refers to as 'authoritative discourse', discourse that is 'indissolubly fused with its authority – with political power, an institution, a person' (p. 343).

Strategies of discourse representation in narratives of illness or recovery function not just to position the narrator in relation to other people in the stories, but also to position the narrator in relation to his or her 'past selves'. This phenomenon is especially evident in stories told by recovering alcoholics, in which the past 'drinking self' is often dramatized through the use of reported speech for the purpose of parody. The following example is from a story told by a fifty-year-old man at an Alcoholics Anonymous meeting.

> When I was 17 years old, I was already into drinking heavily with my friends. One morning we had football practice, and my friends and I were all hung-over. The coach worked us real hard and my friends started falling over and throwing up through their masks. I remember looking at them and feeling sick to my stomach and thinking 'this is madness – this has got to stop!' It was at that moment that I resolved to quit football.
>
> *(Humphreys, 2000, p. 504)*

The juxtaposition of the dramatic and hackneyed direct quotation 'this has got to stop!' with the unexpected resolution that follows highlights the humor of the passage and acts to distance the speaker from the character of his former self. Those who have studied such recovery discourse in detail (see, for example, Cain, 1991; Denzin, 1987; Humphreys, 2000; Jensen, 2000) note that parodying one's own past speech and actions is a common characteristic of such stories. This 'double voicing' of the self is seen as a key stage in the recovery process itself, in which the alcoholic comes to see his or her drinking life as a 'performance that can no longer be played convincingly' (Jensen, 2000, p. 7). Denzin (1987) suggests that alcoholics use humor and self-parody to transcend their past and overcome shame by putting themselves in the position of the laugher rather than the person who is being laughed at.

The multi-voicedness or heteroglossia of narratives, then, like their co-constructed, dialogic aspects, can contribute to their therapeutic power. It allows tellers to reconfigure their experiences through repositioning themselves not just in relation to other people, but also in relation to the selves they used to be, and to take up multiple perspectives, viewing the world and themselves through 'different prisms' (Schiffrin, 1996, p. 169).

*

Throughout this chapter I have been treating inscription and narrativization as two ways of entextualizing the body and, to some extent, have been highlighting the differences between them. At the same time, it should also be clear from the above discussion that these two forms of entextualization are in many ways complementary. In some sense the art of diagnosis can be seen as a process of *resemiotizing* the story the patient tells, and, from the point of view of the patient, a diagnosis is never 'the end of the story', but rather the impetus for further acts of narrativization.

In the next chapter I will consider a different kind of entextualization common in health and risk communication, one in which bodies are turned into artifacts like X-ray and ultrasound images, and how this *virtualization* of the body affects the kinds of actions we can take around health and risk.

7

VIRTUAL BODIES

In March of 2012 a law went into effect in Texas mandating that any woman in the state who seeks an abortion must first undergo an ultrasound. The law also stipulates that while undergoing the procedure the woman must listen to a doctor explain the body parts of the fetus as they appear on the monitor, and after the examination she must sign a document attesting to the fact that she understands what she has seen, which is then placed in her medical file. The law had the strong support of Texas Governor Rick Perry, who declared, 'this important sonogram legislation ensures that every Texas woman seeking an abortion has all the facts about the life she is carrying' (Ertelt, 2012).

The Texas law is not unique. At the time of its implementation similar measures had either been passed or were under consideration in Alabama, Connecticut, Kentucky, Mississippi, Missouri, North Carolina, Oklahoma, Pennsylvania, Rhode Island, South Carolina, Virginia, and West Virginia. Like Governor Perry, the sponsor of the South Carolina bill, Representative Greg Delleney, focused on the informational value of the procedure: 'I'm just trying to ... inform women with the most accurate, non-judgmental information that can be provided,' he said (Fry-Revere, 2007). Pennsylvania Governor Tom Corbett, when asked about the measure being debated in his state, dubbed the 'Woman's Right to Know Act', insisted that the procedure is not intrusive: 'If a woman doesn't want to watch, he said, all she has to do is close her eyes' (Bassett, 2012).

*

Graphic designer Hugo Campos has a US$30,000 cardiac defibrillator (ICD) implanted in his chest to prevent sudden cardiac arrest due to a heart condition he has known as hypertrophic cardiomyopathy. The device collects data about his heart rhythm, his daily activity, variation in chest impedance, as well as information about how many times a day it delivers a shock to his heart muscle, all of which it wirelessly sends to his doctor, who can access it via his iPhone. What concerns Campos is that, although his doctor has constant access to this crucial data about his bodily functions, he himself does not. He can only get it during his visits to his doctor. 'The question,' he declares, 'is who owns this data. I mean here's a device that's part of me, part of who I am, I wake up with it, I go to bed with it, and yet I don't have access to this information' (Campos, 2011).

*

My current weight is 71.8 kg, which is 0.3 kg more than it was yesterday. The percentage of that which is fat is 15.5 percent. My body mass index is 21.8. Whenever I weigh myself, the information is wirelessly uploaded to a website that plots it for me on a graph and automatically 'tweets' it to all those following me on Twitter.

According to the accelerometer that I carry, I took an average of 13,898 steps per day last week, which puts me in the 98th percentile of men my age. During the entire week I travelled 90.66 km and climbed a total of 270 floors. I slept an average of 5 hours 45 minutes per night, which is less than average for men of my age and 6 percent less than the previous week. It took me an average of 11 minutes to fall asleep, and I was awakened an average of 2 times per night.

Last week 40 percent of the average 2,306 calories per day that I took in came from fat – higher than it should be considering the history of heart disease in my family. 19 percent of my calories came from protein, and 41 percent from carbohydrates. I took in an average of 301 mg of cholesterol per day. According to my latest blood work, although my total cholesterol is high (227 mg/dL), my HDL cholesterol (the 'good' kind) is also high (68 mg/dL) and my triglycerides are low (60 mg/dL). My LDL is optimum (118 mg/dL).

My recent genetic test has come back, indicating that I carry a 'G' variant of the single nucleotide polymorphism (SNP) rs6983267 which has been associated with an increased risk of the formation of precancerous adenomatous polyps and the development of colorectal cancer in subjects of European origin. A week after getting the results I bring them to my doctor along with the records of my weight, activity, diet and sleep patterns. 'I think I'm at risk for colorectal cancer,' I tell him.

'Of course you are,' he says. 'You're over fifty and Caucasian.'
'So what can I do?' I ask.
'Have a colonoscopy. You're due for one anyway.'

Concerned that he is not taking my elevated risk seriously enough, I try to explain to him about the G variant of rs6983267, but he hands the genetic report back to me dismissively. 'I don't need this to tell me that you need a colonoscopy. You're over 50 and Caucasian. That's enough.'

*

In this chapter I will discuss a third aspect of bodily entextualization, which I call *virtualization*, a process by which, to use the words of Pierre Lévy (1998, p. 40), 'visible, audible and sensible bodies are multiplied and dispersed outside of us.' Virtualization involves creating artifacts of the body, which can be separated from it in time and space, reconfigured, and recontextualized into different situations.

The three anecdotes above involve different kinds of virtualization: high-tech medical imaging, data gathering by medical devices, and, an increasingly important kind of virtualization, the genetic test. While the form the virtual body takes in all of these examples is different, they all highlight some of the key issues surrounding the entextualization of the body that I brought up in the last chapter, issues of authorship and ownership, issues of what these texts can be used for and what they cannot and by whom, and issues about the personal and political agendas these texts serve.

By virtual bodies I mean all external representations of the body in any mode or media, including drawings, paintings, photography, textual or numerical records of laboratory tests, as well as written or recorded narratives or diagnoses. The virtualization of the human body is not something new. It can be traced back to the early anatomical drawings of the ancient Greeks in the fourth century BC, and even further back to cave paintings of the human form (Jones, 2009a). But it began to become increasingly important in medical practice in the nineteenth century as new technologies for translating the body into texts and images were developed. In the 1860s, for example, the French engineer Etienne-Jules Marey invented an early version of the electrocardiogram (ECG), and in 1895, German scientist Wilhelm Conrad Roentgen invented X-ray photography, allowing the medical gaze new access into the interior of the human body.

Armstrong (1995), drawing on the work of Ackerknecht (1967), argues that the evolution of medicine can be seen in terms of different historical stages, each characterized by where health and illness were *located* in relation to the patient's body. In the seventeenth century, dominated by what he calls 'library medicine', health and illness were located in abstract bodies of knowledge rather than the bodies of individuals. In the eighteenth century, with the development of 'bedside medicine', health and illness were understood as a matter of signs and symptoms on the *surface* of the patient's body. With the advent of 'hospital medicine' of the late eighteenth and nineteenth centuries, spurred on by the invention of tools like the stethoscope that allowed for the investigation of the body's interior, the 'patient's body as a *three-dimensional* object became the focus of medical attention' (Armstrong, 1995, p. 394). In the twentieth century, with the rise of 'laboratory medicine' (Jewson, 1976), the locus of health and illness became the clinical markers derived from laboratory tests and medical images, and in the twenty-first century, with the rise of what Armstrong calls 'surveillance medicine', health and illness have come to be seen as a matter of 'factors' and statistics entirely separate from the physical body. As Armstrong (1995, p. 395) puts it, in the last hundred years, health and illness have left the 'confines ... of the human body to inhabit a novel extracorporal space'. Atkinson (1995, p. 61) makes a similar point when he writes, 'The body of the patient is no longer localized in the discrete integral body of the actual patient. The discursive space of the body is no longer coterminous with the bedside.' Instead, the bedside has become a site where data are collected to generate *virtual* bodies that are dispersed throughout institutions and healthcare systems.

This progressive abstraction of the body from its physical form has been accelerated by the development of digital technology. 'For the first time in history', says cardiologist and geneticist Eric Topol (2012, p. vi), 'we can digitize humans.' Digitizing a human being, he goes on to explain,

> is determining all of the letters ('life codes') of his or her genome ... It is about being able to remotely and continuously monitor each heart beat, moment-to-moment blood pressure readings, the rate and depth of breathing, body temperature, oxygen concentration in the blood, glucose, brain waves, activity, mood ... It is about being able to image any part of the body and do a three-dimensional reconstruction, eventually leading to the capability of printing an organ. Or using a miniature, handheld, high-resolution imaging device that rapidly captures critical information anywhere, such as the scene of a motor vehicle accident or a person's home in response to a call of distress. And assembling all of this information about an individual from wireless biosensors, genome sequencing or imaging for it to be readily available, integrated with all the traditional medical data and constantly updated.
>
> *(Topol, 2012, pp. vi–vii)*

Clarke and his colleagues (2003) use the term *biomedicalization* to describe these changes in the ways human bodies are entextualized, and how those entextualizations are used for the creation of new 'technoscientific identities'. Owing to the rapid technological advances in biomedicine, they point out, the body is no longer regarded as a 'solid', immutable object that can be classified and controlled through processes like inscription and narrativization, but instead has been transformed into something more flexible, capable of being reconfigured and transformed. The focus of bodily entextualization in this new regime of biomedicalization is not on fixing the body, but on 'shifting, reshaping, reconstituting, and ultimately transforming bodies for varying purposes' (Clarke et al., 2003, p. 181).

Virtual bodies have a number of particular characteristics that make this possible. First, they involve a *despatialization* and *detemporalization* of the body, allowing us to decouple it from the physical body. Second, virtual bodies are *reproducible*, and so they can exist in multiple contexts at one time. Third, virtual bodies are always *partial*, with only one or several aspects or 'slices' of the body being revealed, and so virtualization invariably results in a *fragmentation* and dispersion of the body (P. Atkinson, 1995). Finally, precisely because of this process of fragmentation, virtualization allows us (or others) to *reconstitute* our bodies in new ways, to re-create our bodies. As Lévy (1998, p. 44) puts it, virtualization represents 'a recreation, a reincarnation, a multiplication, a vectorization, and a heterogenesis of the human'.

Elsewhere (Jones, 2009b), in theorizing about the virtualization of the body, I have borrowed from Deleuze and Guattari (1987) the notion of 'bodies-without-organs' to refer to the field of possibilities that opens up when humans are able to free themselves from their physical bodies and project themselves across time and space. 'Bodies-without-organs' are dynamic and reflexive, able to be altered and redefined. At the same time, they are also sites of contestation between the individual and the society, which seeks to 'territorialize' them and fix their meaning. Biomedical discourse, as Lupton (2003, p. 24) points out, often tries to territorialize the 'body-without-organs' by transforming it into a 'body-with-organs', making criterial its existence as a set of discrete anatomical structures. Throughout this chapter I will elaborate on this 'double-edged' nature of virtualization, the tension between the ways this form of entextualization opens up new possibilities for the individual for managing his or her own health and risk, and the ways it simultaneously creates new opportunities for institutions and governments to 'territorialize' practices and identities around health.

Medical imaging

In most medical contexts, what we often seem to be dealing with when it comes to virtualization is not 'bodies without organs' but rather 'organs without bodies'. More and more, our experiences with medicine involve the production of high-tech images of our internal organs, which are used to render the body legible to the medical gaze. Different kinds of technologies capture and decontextualize different fragments of the body, which can then be taken away, examined, and resemiotized into diagnoses and treatments. In the century since the invention of X-ray photography, a host of imaging technologies have been developed, including ultrasound, endoscopy, computed tomography ('CT scans'), magnetic resonance imaging (MRI), and positron emission photography (PET).

These new technologies, argues van Dijck (2005), have given rise to a reimagining of the body as 'transparent and knowable', and at the core of this reimagined body, she suggests, are deep-seated cultural notions about progress, rationality, and human perfectibility – in particular the belief that 'seeing' a problem is tantamount to solving it. In a 2010 study Hillman and Goldsmith (2010) attribute what they see as the widespread overuse of medical imaging in part to this underlying belief that 'seeing is curing' (van Dijck, 2005, p. 6). 'The exquisite depictions of anatomy and function generated by modern imaging technologies,' they write, 'have blinded many physicians to the limitations and potential harms of radiologic diagnosis' (p. 5).

While advanced technologies seem to render our bodies more transparent, the reality for most patients is that high-tech scans and other forms of screening create texts which for them are utterly opaque. They must be explained or 'talked into existence' by professionals using highly evolved skills of interpretation and entextualization. Furthermore, physicians are increasingly relying on their analyses of these images and other representations of the body in order to arrive at diagnoses, and their delivery of these diagnoses to patients is increasingly mediated through these artifacts. What this means is that in their interactions, doctors and patients are increasingly oriented not towards each other, but towards external objects as the locus of their attention and discourse.

Virtualization and ideology

Perhaps nowhere are the issues surrounding the role of virtualizations in interactions between doctors and patients more clear than in the routine use of ultrasound imaging on pregnant women. Nowhere, either, is the *ideological* dimension of virtualization more obvious (Stabile, 1992). In the United States and elsewhere, ultrasound images have contributed dramatically to the polarization of opinion not just about biomedical power but also about the meaning of personhood itself (Kevles, 1997).

Ultrasound became widely available for the monitoring of pregnancy in North America and Europe just as the first wave of the feminist movement was at its height, with many women expressing suspicion of the mostly male-dominated medical establishment and asserting the right to 'control their own bodies'. In many ways, ultrasound undermined this assertion, giving to doctors unprecedented power over how the fetus was represented. As van Dijck (2005, p. 106) points out, 'before the invention of ultrasound, pregnancy was primarily considered an individual experience. Only the pregnant woman could feel the fetus moving; outsiders could only hear its heartbeat.' What ultrasonography did was open the woman's womb to the gaze of biomedicine, redefining pregnancy from an 'interior experience' to a 'public event' (Petchesky, 1987).

By the end of the century, ultrasonography had taken on the status of a cultural ritual. Having an ultrasound is now regarded as a defining moment in the pregnancy of most women in the industrialized world (Kevles, 1997), and most hospitals provide patients with pictures or videos of their scans, which become part of photo albums and other artifacts of family history. In many places commercial 'fetal photo studios' have also sprung up, offering ultrasound images packaged as slick DVDs with background music that parents can send to friends and relatives.

Because of this cultural dimension of ultrasonography, it is also usually more interactive than other forms of medical imaging, with patients (and sometimes their spouses or other relatives) often viewing the images along with medical personnel as the procedure is being performed. Indeed this process of 'joint reading' has become extremely important in terms of both the medical and the cultural functions of the scan. As with many other types of medical image, ultrasounds are difficult to interpret without extensive training, and, especially in the early stages of pregnancy, the image may not even be immediately recognizable as a fetus. Parents viewing a scan along with a professional normally wait for the expert's 'permission' before allowing themselves to 'recognize their baby' (van Dijck, 2005, p. 101). In cases where such 'permission' is given, 'it no longer matters if prospective parents really see anything or not – most believe they do' (Kevles, 1997, p. 249).

In other words, healthcare workers use ultrasound images to 'talk the fetal person into existence'. Not only do they help parents discern body parts like the head, limbs, and genitals, but they also interpret various movements in the image as fetal actions. Mitchell and Georges (1997) in their ethnographic study of ultrasound procedures note how medical personnel describe movements on the screen as intentional activities: the fetus 'playing', 'swimming', 'dancing', and 'waving'. They also frequently assign intentions and feelings to the fetus, describing it as 'shy' or 'modest', for example, when visualizing the genitalia is difficult, or 'good' and 'cooperative' when a clear image is attained. Finally, they often address the fetus directly, complementing it, giving it instructions like 'smile for the camera', and even stroking or 'tickling' the onscreen image. This narrativization of the virtual body is even more evident in commercial settings in which the construction of the fetus as a person serves both the emotional needs of customers and the commercial needs of the companies. Roberts (2012) describes a process that she calls 'collaborative coding' in which sonographers and customers work together to construct stories about the fetal person and its relationship to expectant parents. In this process, she argues, not only do professionals assist expectant parents in 'learning to see' the image, but expectant parents contribute their own information about things like family history and their own embodied experience of pregnancy to fill out the picture. In the following excerpt, for instance, the sonographer, the expectant mother, and her male partner work together to construct the fetal activity of thumb-sucking by repeating and expanding on one another's interpretations:

01	Pregnant woman:	Sleepy girl … did she open her eyes then? … wow!
02	Sonographer:	She's settled down again now … see her mouth going?
03		She's got her hands in front of her face … there's a
04		little smile … it's all too much. She's put her thumb in
05		her mouth.
06	Male partner:	She's sucking her thumb (laughing). *(p. 307)*

This 'talking into existence' of the fetal person does not just occur in clinics and commercial ultrasound studios. It is also a regular feature of public discourse. Among the most notorious examples of this is the 1984 film *The Silent Scream*, in which gynecologist turned anti-abortion crusader Dr Benard Nathanson talks the audience through an ultrasound film of the abortion of a twelve-week-old fetus, attributing to the image emotions like fear and confusion and characterizing one moment at which the head of the fetus appears to rear back and its mouth appears to open as the 'child' screaming in pain. It matters little that this assertion is easily disputed by scientific evidence, including the fact that at twelve weeks the fetus has no cerebral cortex to receive pain impulses. The film exploits the natural tendency for viewers of photographs to assign to them an objective reality (Barthes, 1982). This, along with the authoritative narrative of the expert physician, makes it difficult for viewers *not* to see this movement as a scream.

The meaning of virtual bodies, then, is highly contingent and dependent on the practices of *reading* which are constructed in interactions, whether they be interactions between doctors and patients or between onscreen 'experts' and viewers. Just as X-rays and CT scans become mediational means in the construction of diagnoses, ultrasound images in the context of pregnancy become mediational means for the authoring of narratives both at the local level of individual pregnancies, and on the broader cultural level.

The use of ultrasound images in public debates by anti-abortion activists, which began in the 1980s with films like *The Silent Scream*, moved in the 1990s into clinics and doctors' offices under the guise of 'informed consent'. According to the Guttmacher Institute (2012), since the mid 1990s, nineteen US states have adopted some kind of abortion-related ultrasound policy, with six states requiring a woman who wants an abortion to undergo an ultrasound. Although it is not particularly unusual for the state to mandate that people in certain circumstances undergo medical tests, it is unusual for the state to force people to *view* an entextualization of their own body and have that text interpreted for them (Fry-Revere, 2007). The reasons anti-abortion advocates support the use of ultrasound in this way are based mostly on research conducted in the 1980s that suggested that ultrasound images increase the chances of women forming an emotional bond with the fetus (see for example Fletcher and Evans, 1983). Later research, however, has called this assumption into question. Baillie and his colleagues (1999), for instance, found that maternal bonding with the fetus has little to do with the viewing of ultrasound images and more to do with whether or not women have a positive attitude towards their pregnancy to begin with. Studies that support both the theory of maternal bonding and those that call it into question, however, tend to focus only on the *viewing* of the scan and ignore how the represented fetus is *discursively con-structed* in the social interaction among the sonographer, the woman, and the other people present.

Political arguments both for and against state-mandated ultrasonography before an abortion rest on how the process of virtualization is itself framed as a social occasion. Proponents of mandated ultrasounds portray such acts of entextualization as a matter of 'giving information'. This is the framing behind the statements by Governor Perry and Representative Delleney, whom I quoted at the beginning of this chapter, as well as the arguments of the Staff Counsel of the anti-abortion organization Americans United for Life, who writes:

> ultrasound requirements ensure a truly informed choice because they allow a woman to see her unborn child as he or she really is, both by seeing his or her form and face on a screen and also by hearing the heartbeat.
>
> *(Smith, 2012, p. 140)*

While the focus on 'seeing' and 'hearing' in this statement attempts to construct the process of virtualization as unproblematically 'objective', words like 'unborn child' and even 'face' work to create an interpretation of the nature of the object of observation. Moreover, by framing state-mandated ultrasonography as 'information giving', proponents construct women to whom the procedure is administered as 'ignorant' of the 'true nature' of the fetus. This construction represents a shift in popular anti-abortion discourse from depicting women who seek abortions as 'callous, hard, [and] selfish' to depicting them as otherwise 'good' women who are simply 'maternally illiterate' (Hartouni, 1992, pp. 138–39).

Those who oppose mandatory ultrasounds also make use of a 'discourse of rights', but for them what is central is not the 'right to information' but the 'right to privacy'. Thus, instead of framing the act of forcing a woman to undergo an ultrasound as 'information giving', they frame it as an act of *shaming* – 'exposing information' that an individual does not wish exposed. National Organization of Women president Terry O'Neill, for example, characterizes laws requiring women to view an ultrasound before terminating a pregnancy as 'ritual humiliation laws, the intent of which [is] to shame women' (Dolan, 2012). A parody of the Texas law by *Doonesbury* cartoonist Gary Trudeau in March of 2012 depicted a receptionist at an abortion clinic instructing a patient to 'Please take a seat in the shaming room … a middle-aged male state legislator will be with you in a minute' (Trudeau, 2012).

'Shaming' can be seen as a speech act designed to invoke in people a sense of not having lived up to the ethical standards of a community. What is interesting about this speech act is that it is predicated on the process of 'entextualizing the other', normally accomplished through talking about a person in that person's presence (Ochs, 1988). It can involve inscribing a person with some kind of label, or it can involve narrativization, as when parents tell stories about their children when their children are present as a means of socialization (Fung, 1994). It can also involve, as in the case of mandatory ultrasounds, the process of virtualization, creating an image of the target and reflecting that image back at her. In this case, what is made 'visible' is, first of all, the 'potential child', and second of all, the 'potential mother', whose proper role the patient is seen to be failing to fulfill. This process, argues Kumar and her colleagues (2009, p. 5), works to 'expel' the woman seeking an abortion 'from the normative category of "woman"', and this expulsion, they say, has become so much a part of the discourse of abortion in many countries that 'shame' has come to be seen as a 'natural response' to the procedure rather than as socially constructed by the rituals of entextualization that have been set up around pregnancy. 'Today,' writes Løkeland (2004, p. 172), 'it has almost come to the point where you have to say you are sorry and have doubts about your decision to have an abortion in order to be regarded as a moral person.'

My intention here is not so much to decry forced ultrasound laws as to illustrate the fact that the entextualization of the body, no matter how 'scientific' it seems, is never 'objective' and value free. Not only do different processes of entextualization naturally make some aspects of the body criterial and obscure others, but the meaning and significance of these texts are always a matter of how they are appropriated into particular sites of engagement and subjected to the particular agendas and power relationships of those who occupy these sites. Although a sonogram is a type of 'information', the notion that performing an ultrasound is simply an act of 'conveying information' to a patient so that she can make an 'informed choice' grossly simplifies the situation. As Petchesky (1987, p. 287) puts it, 'no image dangles in a cultural void, just as no fetus floats in a space capsule.' 'Treating a fetus as if it were outside a woman's body, because it can be viewed, is a *political* act' (p. 272), made possible by the convergence at particular sites of engagement of certain kinds of social actors and certain kinds of processes of entextualization.

Electronic medical records

Another type of virtual body that frequently intervenes in interactions between doctors and their patients is the electronic medical record. The electronic medical record (rather than the actual body of the patient) is increasingly used as the primary site of clinical decision-making by many healthcare workers. Just as with the constructions of the fetus I described above, which depend on the combination of images with processes of narrativization and inscription, patient medical records are also interdiscursive artifacts in which virtual bodies (images, scans, laboratory tests) are brought together and made meaningful through interaction both between doctors and patients, and among the different healthcare workers who interact with them. Through the processes of entextualization it makes possible, it reconstructs the physical patient as something that is 'manageable' within the scope and routines of the institution and the conceptual boundaries of the various medical specialisms within it. Every act of adding to or modifying it entails an act of 'translation' in which signs, symptoms, stories, and events are *resemiotized* into charts, graphs, tables of figures, coded notes, and other textual objects. These objects impose their own pace and logic upon the patient, with measurements of temperature and pulse being taken at fixed intervals, tests being performed and medicines being administered at times dictated by the record, and observations of the patient undertaken within the set of categories and generic formulae which the record dictates. Through the generic conventions of the record, the patient comes to be rewritten as a 'bureaucratic object' whose rhythms match the shifts of doctors and nurses, the opening hours of laboratories, and the billing procedures of institutions (Berg and Bowker, 1997, p. 519).

Because of the multiple functions medical records perform that are *external* to the actual care and treatment of the patient, they tend to take on a kind of rarified consistency that glosses over the 'messiness' that necessarily characterizes much medical care. Berg and Bowker (1997) note how medical records involve the 'rational reconstruction' of past events in ways that reflect idealized processes of reasoning, which are not always entirely consistent with reality. As the body of the patient is resemiotized into the record, Berg and Bowker write:

> details are omitted, and the story is simplified and retold in ways that fit the present situation at hand. This results in an increasing stylization of past

events into a standard canon: a sign leading to a diagnosis leading to a therapy leading to an outcome.

(p. 525)

This, in turn, they argue, has an effect on the way biomedicine itself is perceived, reinforcing 'master narratives' in which 'patients are cured by doctors' actions; and ... doctors' actions reflect a rational thought process' (p. 525).

Like all texts, electronic medical records serve to construct certain aspects of what they represent as criterial and background other aspects. While few would argue that electronic medical records construct the patient as an efficient *bureaucratic entity*, some believe that they impose obstacles to the construction of the patient as an efficient object of clinical care. In a series of studies, Patel and his colleagues (2000; 2002) found that when physicians were asked to enter the same patient information in both electronic records and handwritten paper records, there was a *loss of information* associated with use of the electronic medical records as compared to paper-based records. One reason for this is that the strict sets of categories and standardized forms of notation in electronic records often make it difficult or impossible to enter certain kinds of information – especially highly individualized information – about patients. Another reason is that electronic records often make it difficult to record how the information was *organized* by the patient as he or she presented it to the doctor, and how the doctor made sense of the temporal flow of the patient's narrative. In the last chapter I pointed out that what is important about patients' narratives is not just their informational content but also how that content is structured in meaningful ways. It is precisely this aspect of patients' narratives that is sacrificed when they are transformed into the standardized categories of electronic medical records. Patel and his colleagues (2002) dramatically illustrate this point by presenting two entextualizations of a patient with a similar complaint, one as part of a paper-based record, and the other as a part of an electronic record. The paper-based record states:

> Patient is 47 years old and is known to be a diabetic for one year, but possibly for longer. He has fatigue, drowsiness, polyuria and nycturia. He was discovered to have diabetes and has been treated by Glucophage and Diabeta since that time. He had an opthamologic evaluation but no renal examination. In 1973 he stepped on a nail, and since that time had 30 operations for repeated infection.
>
> *(p. 13)*

In contrast, the beginning portion of an electronic medical record made by the same doctor about a similar patient reads as follows:

CHIEF COMPLAINT: Type II diabetes mellitus
PERSONAL HISTORY
SURGICAL: cholecystectomy: Age 50 years old

MEDICAL: hyperthyroidism: asymptomatic since 25 years
LIFESTYLE
MEDICATION
DIABETA (Tab 2.5 MG)
Sig: 1 tab(s) Oral before breakfast

The point Patel and his colleagues make is that the first text contains information about the temporal and causal relationships between pieces of information that is obscured in the atomistic way information is treated in the second text. Others have argued that the inability of most electronic medical record systems to accommodate the kind of free-flowing text found on most paper-based records ends up compromising rather than aiding physician decision-making. The problem with electronic records, Walsh (2004) argues, is that they impose not just a one-size-fits-all set of descriptors, but also a one-size-fits-all method of reasoning (based on pattern recognition and hypothetical deductive models), when in many medical encounters clinical decision-making is a more inductive and interactive process of joint narrativization by doctors and patients. In other words, electronic medical records do not just 'aid' in decision-making; they actively promote a certain *kind* of decision-making, one which is couched in the positivist tradition of 'evidence-based medicine'. While this form of decision-making has considerable value, much medical work is also intensely personal, context-bound, and filled with exceptions, and paper records, with their flexibility, portability, and tolerance of ambiguity seem to support this aspect of medical work in ways that electronic record systems, at least those that have been developed to date, cannot (Greenhalgh et al., 2009).

Electronic medical records and the interaction order

Whatever might be said about the ways the discursive features of medical records influence how patients are entextualized and how care and treatment are carried out, none of this can really be understood without attention to how medical records function as a mediational means in actual encounters between doctors and patients, how, for example, they influence concrete interactional features like mutual attention and turn-taking, and how they are used by patients and doctors to claim and impute certain interactional rights and responsibilities.

Studies of such issues from a traditional health communication viewpoint have revealed that the use of electronic medical records has a considerable impact on standard measures of 'successful' doctor–patient communication. Margalit and her colleagues (2006), for example, found that when electronic medical records are used in consultations, doctors spend between a quarter and half of the visit time gazing at the computer screen, and screen-gazing was found to negatively influence physicians' emotional responsiveness. At the same time, however, computer use was found to positively affect information exchange and patient disclosure.

Applied linguists approach such behavior as gaze and keyboarding slightly differently. Rather than simply quantifying such behaviors, they seek to understand how they function at different moments in the encounter to perform different kinds of interactional work. A physician's act of gazing at a computer screen, for example, may serve a number of different functions: it may be a contextualization cue to signal a shift to a new phase or 'frame' (Pearce et al., 2008a); it may function as a claim to expertise, a way for the doctor to demonstrate the practice of 'establishing the facts' (Als, 1997); it may be a way for the physician to indirectly communicate his or her attitude towards what the patient has said; or it may serve as a way for both doctor and patient to take a 'break' in the interaction to reflect on what has been said or to re-establish their bearings (Ventres et al., 2005). Similarly, typing may serve as a way for the physician to 'hold the floor' while recording information, preventing the patient from introducing new topics too quickly; it can serve as a kind of backchannel, a means of signaling to the patient that he or she has been heard and understood; and it can also be used to signal shifts from one line of questioning to a new one (Frankel et al., 2005; Pearce et al., 2008b; Swinglehurst et al., 2011). Patients also make use of the computer as an interactional tool, signaling things like confirmation, uncertainty, and disagreement by gestures like pointing to the computer or adjusting their gaze and posture to either attend to what is being typed or conspicuously dis-attend to it (Pearce et al., 2008b).

One thing that such observations remind us of is that the effect of texts on interactions often has as much to do with the physical properties of those texts as with their discursive properties. Pearce and his colleagues (Pearce, Walker, et al., 2008), for example, note that the placement of the computer screen on the physician's desk can have a significant impact on the way physicians and their patients structure their interactions, with arrangements which allow patients visual access to the screen encouraging more inclusive interactions. In a similar study, however, Winthereik (2004) found that even with the variable of screen direction it is difficult to make generalizations. In some cases, he notes, 'closed screens' can actually foster more patient participation because they can stimulate doctors to translate information from the screen to the patient, while 'open screens' can sometimes result in patients being put off or confused by difficult-to-understand categories and notations.

'Welcome to you!': the reflexive dimension of virtual bodies

Perhaps the biggest problem with most forms of medical virtualization from the patient's point of view is not that they transform them into bureaucratic entities for hospital administrators or that they distract their doctors during consultations, but rather that they themselves often have limited access to them. While in most countries patients have a legal right to obtain copies of things like test results and medical records, the bureaucratic practices of hospitals, laboratories, and medical device companies sometimes make such access difficult (Honeyman et al., 2005). Even when they do obtain their medical records, they usually lack the skills to make sense of them. Furthermore, doctors, until recently, have generally not encouraged patients to access their records, insisting that it might unduly confuse or worry them, or afraid the motivation behind seeking such access might be litigious (Liaw, 1993).

Increasingly, however, patients are taking matters into their own hands, using newly available digital technologies of entextualization not only to access records of their interactions with the healthcare system, but also to create their own textual representations of their health and health behavior. The simplest examples are electronic *personal health records* (PHRs) that patients compile themselves with the help of online tools like Microsoft HealthVault. Much more popular, however, are technologies of entextualization that include a social dimension, allowing users to share their data not just with healthcare professionals but with other users with whom they participate in various kinds of social networks (see next chapter). The technologies also often involve ways for users to automatically upload data using mobile phone applications and sensors such as accelerometers to measure physical activity (like Nike+ for runners) and portable heart rate and blood pressure monitors. Such data might include data about behavior (such as frequency of exercise), about physiology (such as heart rate), or about external conditions that might affect behavior or physiology (such as medical treatments or environment) (Li et al., 2011). According to the Pew Internet and American Life Project (Fox, 2011), one in four US internet users track some aspect of their health information using online tools. Anthropologist J. A. English-Lueck, whose ethnography of the US Silicon Valley contains a detailed description of self-quantification practices among technologically sophisticated young professionals, predicts that, with the proliferation of less expensive and easier-to-use monitoring devices, more and more individuals will begin to engage in self-quantification (English-Lueck, 2010).

In many ways, 'personal informatics', or what has come to be called the 'self-quantification movement' (Mehta, 2011; Wolf, 2010), is a logical outcome of a long historical trajectory in medicine which began with the scientific revolution of the eighteenth century. What characterizes this trajectory is not just a 'trust in numbers' (Porter, 1996), but also an ideological commitment to individualism and self-reliance that is the hallmark of what Scollon and his colleagues (Scollon et al., 2012) call the Utilitarian Discourse System. Its has its roots in Jeremy Betham's 'felicific calculus', an algorithm developed to determine the exact amount of 'happiness' produced by a given social action, as well as the more homespun schemes for self-improvement hatched by the likes of Benjamin Franklin. Self-quantifiers view the self as mutable and perfectible, and the path to this perfection as the careful collection and manipulation of data. Health is seen as 'an equation', as a matter of 'inputs and outputs' (Goetz, 2007). Rose and Novas (2005) have used the term 'digital biocitizenship' to describe the growing trend for individuals to make use of digital technologies to constantly monitor their bodily functions and health behavior. This form of 'citizenship', they write:

> operates within ... a 'political economy of hope.' Biology is no longer blind destiny ... It is knowable, mutable, improvable, eminently manipulable. Of course, the other side of hope is undoubtedly anxiety, fear, even dread at what one's biological future, or that of those one cares for, might hold.
>
> (p. 442)

From a more Foucaultian point of view, self-quantification represents the pinnacle of governmentality, calling upon individuals to take up the task of their own self-governance through a continuous process of self-monitoring and self-improvement (Petersen and Lupton, 1996). It constitutes the logical outcome of what Crawford (1980) calls 'healthism', a neo-liberal ideology which simultaneously elevates health to the status of a moral duty and situates responsibility for it at the level of the individual rather than society.

At the same time there is also a more subversive dimension to this movement that challenges biomedical authority and its control over the means of entextualizing the body. Its extreme form of individualism, in fact, contradicts many of the principles of 'evidence-based medicine' with its emphasis on clinical trials performed on large populations. The gold standard of evidence for self-quantifiers is not the randomized controlled trial, but the unique, unreproducible experience of 'me'. This subversive strain is particularly evident in the rhetoric of 'body hackers' (Ferris, 2010), who advocate extreme programs of self-experimentation and rapid physical modification that many medical professionals would consider ill-advised. Just as early computer hackers borrowed and built upon existing technical systems, body hackers borrow and build upon the tools of biomedicine. The goal, however, is not to fulfill some pre-determined definition of health, but rather to push the limits of the body, to be 'better than well' (English-Lueck, 2010, p. 14).

For applied linguists, what makes the self-quantification movement and other contemporary practices of self-surveillance particularly interesting is the opportunity they present to explore how engaging in the act of entextualization itself affects health behavior and what kinds of discursive features make self-entextualizations effective tools for behavior change. There are a number of ways in which the act of entextualizing the self contributes to health behavior. First, it helps to create for people a sense of agency and feeling of being in control of their reality. In chapter 3 I argued that access to the means of entextualizing reality in part gives one the ability to define it. The relationship between entextualization and self-efficacy has been observed in a wide variety of contexts, from groups like Alcoholics Anonymous where producing various self-entextualizations from personal narratives to lists of one's 'character defects' assists members in managing their recovery from addiction, to online social networking spaces where, as Hull and Katz (2006, p. 69) put it, people create multimedia representations of themselves as a 'means to reposition themselves as agents in and authors of their own lives'. 'Disciplining' the body through acts of self-quantification, argues Frank (1995), is a way for people to compensate for the apparently random and contingent nature of health. There is, however, he warns, a downside to such regimens of self-discipline, in that they can result in self-objectification and isolation.

The way self-quantification works to increase agency is not just by giving people the feeling that they are in control, but by actually making available to them new practices of 'reading' their own bodies that make them more aware of what they are doing and its consequences on their health through creating 'feedback loops' (Goetz, 2010). There is considerable research showing that feedback plays an important role in behavior change (DiClemente et al., 2000), and feedback loops have long been a component of medical treatments for things like pain management. Feedback loops work in two ways: they help people to *discover* trends and patterns in their behavior in order to make plans or set goals for the future, and they help them to *maintain* those plans or advance towards those goals by providing constant information about their progress (Li et al., 2011).

The problem with most health behavior is that the consequences of what we do now are usually not immediately discernible. The negative feedback from smoking a cigarette or eating an extra piece of cake is usually long term and gradual, while the positive feedback is immediate. Similarly, the positive feedback from exercising usually comes long after one experiences the soreness of that first trip to the gym. Self-entextualization serves to create feedback loops that operate on shorter timescales, providing people with more immediate information about their behavior, often tied to some form of reward or punishment, if only an annoying reminder that they have eaten another piece of cake. At the same time, it also allows people to plot long-term trends, to map, for example, their pattern of cake eating over time, on what days and at what times of day it occurs, and what usually 'triggers' it. In other words, self-monitoring creates the opportunity for people to engage with the 'layered simultaneity' (Blommaert, 2005) of their health behavior, reframing or 're-circumferencing' the way they experience their behavior and their body's response to it. Many technologies of self-entextualization allow users to check on their immediate status at any given moment, to take a retrospective view of their behavior over time, to set goals for future behavior, and to relate behavior at any given time with the contexts in which it occurred or the factors which may have influenced it.

Another important factor in understanding the utility of self-entextualization for behavior change is the way processes of entextualization themselves are able to make criterial aspects of people's physiology or behavior which they find relevant. Technologies people use for self-quantification *resemiotize* data on health states or actions into durable textual artifacts that give these states and actions new meaning. The data sent from my Wi-Fi scale is converted into a graph that illustrates my weight loss or gain over time. The website for Nike+ maps my run and allows me to choose any location on the map to find out how fast I was going at any given moment. It also allows me to compare my performance to other people of my age and gender, or to myself on other days, or to the goals that I have set for myself. Most technologies for self-quantification make use of information visualization techniques (Card et al., 1999) that transform temporal or quantitative information into spatial information, allowing people to 'see' trends over time or to easily compare two or more quantities. Frost and Smith (2003), for example, show how using multimodal texts can help diabetic patients explore the relationship between their blood glucose level and the types of food they consume. The software they developed displays the information in a variety of graphical ways that facilitate patients' moving up and down different timescales, from a simple 'timeline' in which photographs of meals patients have taken with their mobile phones appear next to blood glucose measurements, to a historical grid in which recorded glucose values appear as colored squares indicating how close the readings are to recommended target ranges. Each square in the grid is also hyperlinked, allowing users to move easily from the historical overview to particular moments in the timeline. This combination of semiotic modes, the authors argue, helps users to make connections between their physiological measurements and their behavioral routines.

A final important feature of many of these texts that seems to make them effective tools for behavior change is that they are *shared* with others. As I have shown above, more traditional entextualizations of the body in medical contexts have an important social dimension, with patients or physicians displaying and interpreting textual bodies in various forms to each other. Digital media make it possible to engage in these acts of display and interpretation with a much larger number of people. Broadcasting, discussing, and comparing one's self-entextualizations with others (who are not necessarily professionals) turns health into a *social* activity, mitigating the 'monadic' isolation which Frank (1995) saw as a danger of self-discipline. Sharing information with people who reciprocate by sharing their own information gives one a sense of social connectedness, and others' reactions and comments function to enhance the efficiency of feedback loops.

Related to this social dimension of self-quantification is the way many self-tracking technologies work to transform health-related practices into 'entertainment'. The Fitbit website awards me a 'badge' every time I climb a certain number of stairs and transmits that fact to my Facebook wall, and the Nike+ website allows me to 'race' with my friends, whether we are running at the same time or not. This 'gamification' of health practices (Dembosky, 2011) not only increases motivation, but also contributes to learning. In his book *What Video Games Have to Teach Us about Learning and Literacy*, James Gee (2003) explores video games from the perspective of 'New Literacy Studies'. The qualities he associates with video games that are successful in engaging players in a process of rapid and effective learning are also characteristics of many of the most popular technologies people use for self-tracking, including interactivity, the ability to customize and personalize the experience, the provision of 'just in time' information, and the presentation of information in multiple modes (audio, visual, textual, and tactile) to make the learning experience more 'embodied' (p. 48). Ironically, when it comes to understanding the consequences of our health behavior, the actual body is often a poor mediational means; 'virtual bodies' that represent our bodily experiences in the form of text, images, and audible 'alerts' (like 'cheers' when we run an extra kilometer) can contribute to making information about our bodies *feel* more 'embodied'.

Personal genomics and the entextualized body

Perhaps the ultimate capacity to entextualize the body came with the successful sequencing of the human genome at the dawn of the millennium. Technological advances since then, which have made genomic analysis progressively cheaper, have brought this means of entextualization within reach of private customers. For between US$300 and US$1000, individuals can submit a tissue sample for DNA analysis to businesses like DecodeMe, Navagenics, and the one I used for my own genetic test, the Silicon Valley company 23andMe, and receive a detailed report on disease risks, carrier status, ancestry, and a host of other genetically influenced traits, unmediated by the expert advice of a physician or genetic counselor. Some services also give customers ways to interact with and share their genetic information with other customers via *Facebook*-style social media platforms and to participate in medical research.

These services, of course, are not without their critics. While personal genomics companies claim that direct-to-consumer genetic testing helps people to make healthy lifestyle choices, skeptics assert that such tests can lead to undue anxiety and unnecessary medical procedures (Kutz, 2010; McGuire and Burke, 2011). Others point to the low clinical validity of such testing in its current form, labeling it 'recreational genomics' and even comparing it to astrology (van Ommen and Cornel, 2008). Finally, many insist that laypeople lack the requisite expertise to interpret the results of genetic tests, that such tests are at best useless and at worst dangerous without the intervention of a professional to 'read' them for their patients. In a letter to the U.S. Food and Drug Administration, the American Medical Association (2011) expressed 'concerns that the unfettered and unregulated growth of genetic tests marketed directly to consumers will have a significant adverse impact on consumers and undermine the physician–patient relationship'. The letter also warned that such testing 'in many cases ... represents the unauthorized practice of medicine'.

Whatever the validity or utility of such tests, personal genomics nevertheless has already had an impact on the way people think about the relationship between health and identity (Levina and Quinn, 2011). Genomics has long been used as 'a technology of identity fabrication' (Hauskeller, 2006, p. 3), serving as evidence of paternity, ethnicity, ancestry, normality, carrier-status, health, and even guilt and innocence in criminal trials. The way personal genomics services are marketed to the public further promotes this link between genetics and personal identity. Even the names of the leading personal genomics companies, with their appropriation of different forms of the first person personal pronoun – such as 23and*Me*, deCODE*me*, Kno*me*, *My*cellf, and *My*genome – advance a view of personal genomics as essentially a means of discovering one's 'true self'. 23andMe's website promises to help users 'take a bold, informed step toward self-knowledge', and when I log onto my account, I am greeted with the words 'Welcome to you!'

Like the 'child' in ultrasound images, however, the 'you' in commercial genetic tests does not exist in the 'data' itself, but must be 'talked into existence' in the ways these companies interact with their customers, and, as with prenatal ultrasounds, these discursive processes end up raising broader questions about power, expertise, ethics, and ultimately, what it means to be a person. As Sarangi (2000) has noted, even in professional settings, talking about genetic tests is a complex, 'hybrid' activity that draws upon different discourse types and involves doctors, nurses, and genetic counselors and their clients in complex discursive negotiations about 'what they are doing' and 'who they are being'. Commercial personal genomics involves potentially even more complex and contentious negotiations as companies simultaneously position themselves as marketers selling a product, as medical professionals offering advice, as scientists conducting research, and as political crusaders championing people's 'right to know'.

These multiple positions give rise not just to discursive complications for the companies, but also legal ones. Part of the attraction for users of personal genomics testing services, for example, is that they provide what is construed as a medical service: diagnosing people's chances of contracting certain diseases or medical conditions. This assumption is reinforced by the 'discourse of risk' (Rainville, 2009) that pervades the communication between these companies and their customers. 23andMe, for example, calculates customers' 'disease risks' by matching their genetic variants (single nucleotide polymorphisms) with the findings from hundreds of genome-wide association studies (GWAS) and then summarizes these risks in the form of various graphs and pictorial representations. For most customers, of course, these 'at-risk' identities do not constitute actual conditions. Although I am 'at risk for colorectal cancer', I do not presently have it (according to the colonoscopy I just got), and I may never get it. The way risk is constructed on these sites, however, is as a *trait* of individuals rather than a set of abstract mathematical probabilities. This positioning of customers as 'pre-symptomatic patients' (Levina and Quinn, 2011, p. 2) is, of course, part of a larger trend in medicine of redefining disease in terms of future possibilities rather than present symptoms. Personal genomics accelerates this trend. Although most of these sites are careful to mention that such calculations of risk do *not* constitute diagnoses, most customers believe they do. In a study of the attitudes and beliefs of people who have used personal genomic testing, McGuire and his colleagues (2009) found that 60 percent of their sample considered the information obtained from their test to be a diagnosis of medical conditions or diseases.

What is problematic about this construction is that those who operate such services, by and large, are *not* medical practitioners and so are, in most cases, legally prohibited from issuing diagnoses or offering other forms of medical advice. Consequently, like the genetic counselors in Sarangi's work (2000; Sarangi and Clarke, 2002), the companies need to carefully negotiate their positions to avoid explicitly giving medical advice while at the same time preserving their positions as 'experts'. This is not always easy. In fact, in the same letter to the FDA which I quoted from above, the American Medical Association (2011) comes close to accusing personal genomics companies of outright deception:

> Companies have stated that their tests are not intended to be diagnostic in nature, yet results are presented to patients as an increase/decrease in risk for developing certain conditions. We argue that this is, in fact, diagnostic, especially to consumers seeing these results without the benefit of a health care professional to explain what they mean. This is the unauthorized practice of medicine and should be prohibited.

Interestingly, the techniques companies use to escape such accusations are in many ways similar to those which Sarangi (2000) points out genetic counselors use to avoid being regarded by their clients as purveyors of medical advice. The chief technique is to reframe what they are doing as 'information giving' rather than advising. In an interview with author Thomas Goetz, for example, the CEO of 23andMe Anne Wojcicki insisted that 23andMe's results are not a diagnosis, but rather 'simply *your* information'. This framing of the results as 'information' gives the impression that the construal of disease risk is purely a matter of interpretation by the client (although the language on the 23andMe website pretty much guarantees this construal). Moreover, by using the possessive pronoun *your*, Wojcicki gives the impression that the information is not created by the company, but rather somehow 'naturally existing' in the customer. All the company is doing is restoring it to its 'rightful owner'.

Another technique companies use to deny responsibility for the arguably 'medical' nature of their activities is to hedge and offer disclaimers of various kinds. In their Terms of Service, for example, 23andMe (2012c) reminds customers that:

> The genetic information provided by 23andMe is for research and educational use only … The Services Content is not to be used, and is not intended to be used, by you or any other person to diagnose, cure, treat, mitigate, or prevent a disease or other impairment or condition, or to ascertain your health … 23andMe does not recommend or endorse any specific course of action, resources, tests, physicians, drugs, biologies, medical devices or other products, procedures, opinions, or other information that may be mentioned on our website.

Such disclaimers are often relegated to separate sections of the companies' sites (such as 'Terms of Service' or 'Privacy Statement'), and the interpersonal resources of entextualization they draw on tend to be very different from those used in more 'consumer oriented' sections. Whereas most of the 23andMe website, for example, makes use of frequent personal pronouns ('you' to describe their customers and 'we' or 'us' to describe the company), conversational language (including rhetorical questions and imperatives), and active voice constructions, disclaimers tend to be written in the 'social language' of the law, with the company referring to itself in the third person, using formal language, and making frequent use of the passive voice.

Finally, like the genetic counselors in Sarangi's studies, personal genomics companies are often careful to delineate 'zones of expertise', directing users to third parties to get advice or help in interpreting the information they have provided. The 23andMe website includes in its Terms of Service the instruction to 'always seek the advice of your physician or other appropriate healthcare professional with any questions you may have regarding diagnosis, cure, treatment, mitigation, or prevention of any disease or other medical condition or impairment or the status of your health' (23andMe, 2012c), and in the presentation of risk profiles for various diseases they provide lists of resources such as support organizations or medical websites with disease-specific information.

There is, then, a kind of double voicedness that personal genomics companies make use of to negotiate their positions *vis-à-vis* their customers and the services they are providing. On the one hand, they insist that the information is purely for educational purposes and what they are doing has nothing to do with providing a medical service. These claims, however, are undercut by the presentation of the information in terms of medical risks and clinical usability (Rainville, 2009). In fact, the words 'risk' (as in 'risk calculator', 'health risk', 'disease risk', and 'genetic risk') and 'clinical' (as in 'clinical trials', 'clinical guidelines', 'clinical practice', and 'clinical utility') are among the most frequently used words on the 23andMe website.

At the same time, the claims by critics of such companies that they are 'practicing medicine without a license' is also highly problematic, governed by old assumptions about technologies of entextualization and medical record keeping that no longer function in the age of self-quantification and the 'digital human' (Topol, 2012). New forms of self-entextualization are 're-technologizing' social practices like 'medical testing' and remapping the 'zones of expertise' within which commercial entities, customers, and medical professionals can position themselves. As Prainsack and her colleagues (2008, p. 34) point out in a commentary in *Nature*:

> The California Department of Public Health, when sending cease-and-desist letters to several personal-genomics companies, assumed that a medical test is a distinct entity governed by a clearly discernible set of experts: doctors and public-health authorities. This no longer holds true. Genomics blurs the boundaries that make such clear distinctions possible. A genome scan reveals information that is medical, genealogical and recreational. And those who scan and interpret the data are not distinct bodies of experts, but instead, novel configurations of geneticists, customers, ethicists, bioinformatics experts and new media executives.

Another area in which personal genomics companies must carefully negotiate their relationships with their customers regards the use of customers' genetic information for research purposes. As with other social networking services, the customers of companies like 23andMe are not just customers – they are also, in a very real sense, the 'products' of these companies. The business model of 23andMe and companies like it depends not just on selling personalized genetic risk information to individuals, but also on establishing a database of genetic, phenotypic, and lifestyle information which can be used for research by universities, private laboratories, and pharmaceutical companies. Managing customers' understanding of how their personal information is being used and securing their 'informed consent' can be tricky, especially since the protocols for informed consent in medical research and principles regarding the ownership of human tissue are already fraught with ethical questions.

One way these companies 'sell' participation in research activities to their customers is to discursively construct for them an 'active' role in these activities, labeling them, as 23andMe does, 'collaborators', 'advisers', and 'contributors'. In reality, while customers can sometimes make suggestions about research and how it is conducted in 'community' discussion groups, most of their collaboration, advice, and contributing consists solely of relinquishing information, both in the form of their DNA, and in the form of answers to hundreds of personal questions about their lifestyle, medical history, and family members. One thing that makes this level of 'sharing' palatable to customers is the reframing of their consent as a matter of enlightened self-interest (Tutton and Prainsack, 2011). This entrepreneurial dimension of participation is promoted through the use of metaphors from the language of finance: '23andMe', for example, explains how giving consent for their data to be used for research purposes 'gives customers the opportunity to leverage their data by contributing it to studies of genetics' (23andMe, 2012b). As Tutton and Prainsack (2011, p. 1090) note:

> In the case of 23andMe, we see the construction of the 'enterprising self' who is addressed through a discourse of democratization and empowerment, and who has the right to information as a value in itself. This 'enterprising self' is willing to pay for information about personal genetic risks while, at the same time, will also actively contribute towards new research. Rather than being an altruistic 'gift-giver', [the] participant is engaged in a consumer transaction by which she both purchases and provides information about herself.

Much of how companies like 23andMe get customers to give them valuable information, however, has less to do with positioning them as 'research collaborators' or 'enterprising consumers' and more to do with positioning them as part of a *social network*, the very existence and structure of which compels them to engage in acts of 'sharing'. 'By "sharing" your genome with other … customers,' says the 23andMe website (2012b), 'you can trace shared ancestry, get a glimpse of the diversity in different people's genetics, or simply brag about how you're more Neanderthal than your friends.' Levina and Quinn (2011) argue that the entire enterprise of personal genomics, as with many other web 2.0 enterprises, depends upon constructing the individual as 'a constant stream of information to be shared with other individuals in the network' (p. 2). The benefits customers gain from the service come not just from gaining access to their own genetic information, but from the new social relationships made possible by this information. One's genetic information becomes a form of social capital which one can spend interacting with others, building various alliances, cultivating ties, and trading social identities.

As with Facebook and other social networking sites, 23andMe's site comes with a variety of technologies of entextualization that facilitate and encourage the sharing of information. Customers, for example, are introduced to 'relatives' (usually fourth or fifth cousins, of whom each of us has thousands) and invited to 'share their genes' with them. They are encouraged to become part of various discussion groups or 'communities' with interest in particular diseases or conditions. And they are asked constantly to complete surveys with playful names like 'Ten Things About You', 'Just a Little Bite', and 'The Eyes Have It'. This gamification of information giving, just as with the gamification of self-quantification I discussed above, helps to motivate customers to participate, but it can also serve to distract them from the fact that they are giving away a great deal of personal information about themselves.

Also, as with Facebook, customers are encouraged to share data about themselves partly by being made to see themselves as 'individuals' with unique traits that are 'worth sharing'. The language of individualism pervades the discourse of personal genomics companies. As the website for Navigenics (Navigenics, 2012), for example, announces to customers: 'You're one of a kind. Your health should be too.' Rainie and Wellman (2012) call this brand of individualism in which one's place in the network is justified by one's 'specialness', and one's 'specialness' is reinforced by one's identity as a node in a network *networked individualism.*

While on their websites 23andMe and companies like it construct their customers as 'special' and 'unique' people, and as enlightened 'collaborators' in cutting-edge research, in other research-related contexts they construct them quite differently. In its submission to an independent ethical review board preceding the publication of what they characterized as a 'participant-driven study' of twenty-two genetically influenced traits (Eriksson et al., 2010), for example, 23andMe applied for an exemption from review on the basis that their activity did *not* constitute research on 'human subjects'. Their argument was basically that they were conducting research on entextualized bodies rather than 'real' ones, that they had, in fact, never had actual contact with any of the 'real' people from whom this information was obtained. Based on the technical criteria of the United States Department of Health and Human Services on what constitutes 'research on human subjects' – that investigators obtain the data through intervention or interaction with participants, and the identity of the subjects can be readily ascertained by investigators – the review board agreed with the company that their research did not involve human subjects. In other words, for the purposes of obtaining the data, participants are constructed as real-life individuals, 'collaborators', and 'advisors', while for the purposes of gaining ethical approval, they are constructed as merely 'texts' (Gibson and Copenhaver, 2010).

Much of the success these companies have in negotiating these multiple relationships with their customers depends upon their underlying promotion of a neo-liberal ideology whose primary values include freedom, autonomy, egalitarianism, and the right to private property. The 'ideal customer' of companies like 23andMe is the 'free and creative individual' of the writings of Locke, Bentham, and Mill (Scollon et al., 2012). In fact, one of the most pervasive and persuasive arguments personal genomics companies make to potential customers is that by knowing about their genetic susceptibility to various diseases and medical conditions, they can increase their personal freedom and the range of choices that are available to them, and that access to such knowledge is not a privilege, but a 'right'. 'Freedom to explore one's own biology, all the way down to the molecular level,' writes Jason Bobe (2008) on the influential personal genomics blog *The Personal Genome,* 'should be among the freedoms we hold dear as individuals.'

By framing personal genomics in a discourse of 'rights' and 'freedom', proponents of personal genomics transform their argument with critics from a medical one to a political one. In response to FDA concerns that an unregulated genomic testing industry might actually create health hazards, for example, 23andMe asserted that, while they are 'sensitive to the FDA's concerns,' they 'believe that people have the *right* to know as much about their genes and their bodies as they *choose*' (Pollack, 2010, emphasis mine). This same argument is narrativized in a 'testimonial' on the company's website by a customer named Carole Kushnir entitled 'Don't stand between me and my DNA' (23andMe, 2012a). The story relates how when this 'former grade school teacher and a savvy entrepreneur' read 'a comment from a prominent Stanford professor, who questioned the value of using a person's DNA to determine their genetic risk for diseases, she took it personally'.

> 'It assumes a dumb consumer,' said Carole, who owns a chain of hair salons with her husband, a retired physicist.
> She thought that just didn't add up and didn't give people credit for having common sense. It also ignores the possibility of good outcomes like bringing to a person's attention an unknown risk. That's what happened to her.

The story goes on to relate how Carole purchased a genetic test from 23andMe and found out that she was at risk for breast and ovarian cancer, prompting her to consult with her doctor and eventually to elect to have laparscopic surgery to have her ovaries removed.

> The value of the test was pretty clear to Carole – it detected a risk for cancer she never expected. It prodded her to discuss that possible risk with her doctor and a genetic counselor.
> What wasn't so clear for her is why giving people access to their own genetic information has drawn so much criticism.
> 'Today, more than ever, [information is] important to not only treat disease but to identify those at risk who can then make informed decisions to prevent disease,' she said.

This story and others like it on sites for personal genomics companies illustrate the ways such companies strategically exploit the 'storyline' of the clash between the 'common sense' 'voice of the lifeworld' and the bureaucratic and elitist 'voice of medicine', the very same storyline appropriated by the anti–vaccination activists I discussed in chapter 3. New media technologies like the mobile internet and Web 2.0, with their ethos of open information and mass participation, further fuel this storyline, giving 'ordinary people' the means to access medical information without the help of experts and to display their 'lay expertise' to others online.

*

In the last two chapters I have considered the different ways the body is entextualized in various domains of health and risk, and the different affordances and constraints these texts impose on how people are able to think and communicate about their actual bodies, participate in social practices, and claim and impute social identities. Some of these forms of entextualization, like narrativization, are familiar to applied linguists, whereas others, such as those associated with what Topol (2012) calls the 'digitization of the human', like genetic tests and electronic medical records, may be less familiar. The challenge for applied linguists is to go beyond the structure and meaning of such texts to understanding their role in mediating social actions and social identities and organizing social practices and social organizations.

One of the recurring themes of the last two chapters has been the way in which power relationships affect how bodies are entextualized and the kinds of social actions these texts can be used to take. The technologies of entextualization available to patients for entextualizing their own bodies (chiefly narratives) and those available to doctors and other medical personnel (including diagnosis, and an array of high-tech virtualization techniques) come with different kinds of affordances and constraints and allow their users to claim different degrees of power and types of expertise. One of the most important points I made, however, is that all entextualizations of the body are to some degree jointly authored: laypeople and professionals co-construct illness narratives, collaborate in formulating diagnoses, and work together to interpret things like medical scans and genetic tests.

Recently, new technologies of entextualization have altered the discursive balance of power, putting patients more in control of creating entextualizations of their own bodies and of using them to interact in a range of different social situations that may or may not include medical professionals. Some see these new technologies as ushering in a new era in 'patient-driven' healthcare characterized by 'transparency, customization, collaboration and choice' (Swan, 2009, p. 492; see also Goetz, 2010). Others, however, have pointed out how these new technologies can just as easily be used to promote regulation, bureaucratization, commodification, and exploitation of people's bodies. The challenge for applied linguists is in understanding how practices of 'reading' and 'writing' bodies in different contexts by different kinds of people affect how things like power, control, expertise, and health itself are constructed, negotiated, contested, and controlled.

Textual bodies, like all texts, take their meanings from the situations into which they have been appropriated and the uses to which they are put within particular communities, professions, and institutions, where members share particular conventions and assumptions about 'reading' and 'writing' such texts. At the same time, textual bodies can also serve as 'boundary objects' (Star and Greisemer, 1989), interfaces between multiple communities, professions, and institutions, facilitating the flow of information and resources and the formation of social ties. In the next chapter I will explore how different forms of social organization – communities, 'cultures', institutions, and social networks – affect the way texts about health and risk are produced, circulated, appropriated and resisted, and how texts about health and risk themselves function to create and maintain social groups.

8

CULTURES, COMMUNITIES, AND SOCIAL NETWORKS

In his book *Ethics in an Epidemic: AIDS, Morality and Culture* (1994), Timothy Murphy relates a surprising experience he had when teaching a course on 'AIDS and Ethics' at Beijing Medical University in the early 1990s. During a classroom activity in which his Chinese students role-played a committee of hospital administrators formulating a policy for healthcare workers diagnosed with HIV, Murphy found that the opinions they put forth sounded remarkably familiar. 'As I listened to the Chinese students,' he marvels, 'I was struck time and time again by their raising of many of the issues that surfaced as concerns during [our own] committee meetings; many of the same recommendations were advanced and many of the same criticisms of those proposals emerged' (p. 120).

Later in the same course, however, Murphy's beliefs about how similar the Chinese are to 'us' are shaken when his students uniformly identify kissing as a route of HIV transmission. 'My effort to correct the impression that kissing could cause HIV infection was met with skepticism,' he recalls. 'I even told one physician from a rural province that I myself had kissed people with HIV. "Why would you kiss someone with AIDS?" he asked, shocked, shaking his head as much in warning as disbelief.' Based on this incident, Murphy comes to the conclusion that the belief that HIV is highly communicable 'may be a cultural perception difficult to extinguish' (pp. 123–24).

*

In North America and Europe many heterosexuals still regard AIDS as a 'gay disease', a fact reflected in low rates of condom use among young heterosexual couples, who see themselves as invulnerable to infection. One young man interviewed for a 2003 study (Flood, 2003, p. 364) put it this way: 'In the heterosexual community it's pretty rare that you'll catch a disease ... clean sex acts, in just normal circumstances, very low chance of catching something.'

In many countries in Africa and Asia, the situation is different. There, it is often gay men who see themselves as immune to HIV. In a study of gay men's attitudes towards AIDS in Addis Ababa, for instance, Tadele (2010) found a widespread belief that AIDS is exclusively a heterosexual disease. 'I don't believe zegoch [an idiom for gay men] can get HIV,' one of his participants told him, 'since they only go out with guys.' 'I think it is more risky to have sex with a woman,' another said. 'I don't think it is transmitted that much through unprotected male-to-male sex.' I found similar attitudes during my own fieldwork among men who have sex with men in China in the late 1990s. 'Here in China,' one of my contacts told me, 'we think drug addicts and prostitutes are the ones who get AIDS. "Comrades" [an idiom for gays and lesbians] don't get it' (Jones, 2002a, p. 397).

*

During the summer of 1999, a syphilis outbreak occurred in San Francisco among gay men who used an American Online chat room called SFM4M to find sexual partners. City health authorities linked the infections of seven patients who had tested positive for syphilis in public clinics to an overlapping social network of ninety-nine recent sexual partners who used the same online service (Ornstein, 2002).

The episode was a pivotal event in health officials' understanding of the potential of the internet to contribute to the spread of infectious diseases. Subsequent research has found that an important aspect of this potential is the power of online social networks to facilitate not just the spread of viruses and other pathogens (by making it easier for people to establish 'real life' contact), but also to facilitate the spread of *behaviors* that put people at risk for infection (see for example Bull, 2001; Halkitis and Parsons, 2003; McFarlane et al., 2000).

At the same time, online social networks also have the potential to help healthcare workers trace the spread of epidemics and promote healthy behaviors. Christakis and Fowler (2010), for example, have created a Facebook app which analyzes newsfeed data to predict an individual's risk of getting the flu on any given day, and social networking sites like PatientsLikeUs allow people suffering from various diseases to share and aggregate data about things like symptoms, test results and treatments. Even in the San Francisco syphilis epidemic of 1999, the internet was instrumental in helping public health officials track and notify the sexual partners of infected men and contain the epidemic (Klausner et al., 2000).

*

Throughout this book I have been emphasizing the fact that health and risk are not just a matter of individual choices, but rather are discursively constructed within social groups. These groups come in many shapes and sizes. For most of us, of course, the most important group is our family, but there are other important groups as well: groups that form around certain kinds of activities that may impact our health such as drug taking or extreme sports, professional groups like those of doctors, nurses and health promoters, institutions like hospitals and insurance companies, social networks that connect us through complex webs of relationships to people we do not know and may never meet, and those often rather amorphous groups that we refer to as 'cultures'. All of these groups can have an enormous impact on how we think, talk, and act around health and risk, and the ways we think, talk, and act about health and risk can also function as tools for maintaining these groups and constructing boundaries between them (Douglas and Wildavsky, 1982).

Thinking about health and risk in terms of social structures like 'cultures', 'communities', and 'social networks', however, can be problematic, first because people participate in such groups in a variety of ways, sometimes as full-fledged 'members' and sometimes on the peripheries, and second because we all participate in many different groups at one time: we are simultaneously members of families, professions, interest groups, cultures and nations, and the way we talk and act about health and risk is often a matter not of our participation in any one group but of the ways we manage the boundaries between these intersecting and overlapping groups.

The examples above illustrate some of the issues regarding cultures, communities, and social networks I will address in this chapter. The initial surprise of Professor Murphy, in the first example, that people from such a 'different culture' as the Chinese could hold the same beliefs and values as Americans about AIDS, and his subsequent readiness, when they were found to hold different (i.e. 'wrong') beliefs, to attribute them to 'cultural perceptions', is typical of many discussions about culture and health. Beliefs, attitudes, and behaviors that are just like ours are considered 'natural', and those that are different, particularly those that are radically so, are labeled 'cultural'. With increased migration and globalization, intercultural communication has become a major preoccupation in healthcare, and has also been an area in which applied linguists have contributed important insights (see for example Roberts, 2006). Approaches which essentialize culture and uncritically assign beliefs and behaviors to people based on their 'culture', however, can sometimes end up distorting rather than clarifying our analyses of health-related interactions.

The second example shows how perceptions of group membership sometimes function as what Mendés-Leite (1998) calls 'imaginary protections', feelings of invulnerability to certain health risks based on group affiliation. Ironically, such feelings can sometimes lead to behaviors (like unsafe sex) that actually make these people *more* vulnerable to the very risks they believe themselves immune to. It is easy to dismiss such feelings as a matter of ignorance and prejudice. Sometimes, however, they serve important functions for these groups, functions which are not always evident to health promoters, like creating solidarity, strengthening group identity, and countering discriminatory attitudes or policies from other, more powerful groups.

The final example illustrates how diseases and the health behaviors that cause them are spread through social networks that can extend beyond traditional group boundaries. The importance of social networks in the spread of contagion has long been a preoccupation of epidemiologists and public health officials (see for example Langlie, 1977). The internet, with the new patterns of social interaction and forms of discourse it makes possible, has in some ways facilitated the rapid spread of both pathogens and of health-related ideas, attitudes, and behaviors. Understanding how health and risk communication operates within and across social networks, whether online or offline, with their complex webs of connections, can pose a particular challenge for applied linguists accustomed to analyzing 'focused interactions' (Goffman, 1966) and discrete 'speech communities' (Hymes, 1974).

'Culture' and health

Of all of these forms of social organization, none is discussed in relation to health and risk more frequently than 'culture'. The past half-century has seen a prodigious accumulation of literature in anthropology, sociology, and social psychology on the relationship between health and 'culture' (see for example Ahmad, 1993; Donovan, 1984; Kleinman, 1988; Kreps and Kunimoto, 1994).

The emphasis on 'culture' in studies of health and risk has in part been a reaction to the methodological individualism that has characterized much mainstream medical and health promotion discourse (Fishbein and Middlestadt, 1989; see chapter 5). Approaches to health and risk that trade in the individual as a unit of analysis in favor of notions like 'culture', however, are not without their own problems. To begin with, in many such approaches 'cultures' are seen as either bounded entities, things that people 'live inside of' or as things people possess like property, ignoring the ways individuals strategically pick and choose among a complex and sometimes contradictory array of social practices and social identities when interacting. With the rise of globalization and an increase in the variety of cultural resources available to people to take action around health and risk, talk of stable and discrete 'cultures' becomes even more problematic. In her ethnography of health behavior in California's Silicon Valley, J. A. English-Lueck (2010) notes how most of the people she met engaged in a radically eclectic 'medical pluralism', drawing on traditions as diverse as high-tech body monitoring (see chapter 7), yoga, Chinese acupuncture, and New Age 'energy work'. Such shifting assemblages of cultural resources, she notes, are fast becoming the norm in developed countries, and even in the developing world 'modern' allopathic medicine often exists in complementary ways with older, more indigenous approaches. Under these circumstances, she asks, 'Is culture really relevant anymore, or is it only a placeholder for the constantly morphing identities of people who happen to connect?' (p. 32).

Faced with these theoretical challenges, applied linguists put forth a more modest but in some ways more practical definition of culture. Cultures are seen not as systems of belief or behavior, but as 'systems of discourse' (Scollon, et al., 2012), resources that people have at their disposal to discursively construct various social practices and social identities and to enact those practices and claim those identities in situated social interactions. While intercultural miscommunication around health and risk is sometimes the result of people holding different beliefs about things like the workings of the body and the mechanisms of contagion, it is perhaps more often a matter of them holding different beliefs about the workings of discourse: about how different aspects of health and risk should be *represented*, about who is supposed to say what to whom, when, where, and how, and about the ways texts and conversations should be structured. Even when things like attitudes and beliefs do affect the ways people communicate about health and risk, applied linguists are likely to see them not as static 'sets of assumptions', but rather as part of 'active *discourses*' (Roberts, 2010, p. 216, emphasis mine) which people draw upon strategically to take action and claim identities in specific situations.

Applications of this perspective generally take one of two analytical approaches, either focusing on the ways people from different groups manage interactions around health and risk with respect to things like framing, positioning, and conversational management, an approach which draws heavily on insights from interactional sociolinguistics, or focusing on broader aspects of discourse (including things like ideologies, face systems, and cultural conceptions of the self and communication) and how people draw on them in order to achieve certain interactional goals, an approach which draws on linguistic anthropology.

Interactional sociolinguistics focuses on the fact that people from different groups sometimes bring to interactions different expectations about the moment-by-moment metacommunicative management of 'what they are doing' and 'who they are being' (Gumperz, 1982; Tannen, 2005). People may enter into interactions around health and risk, for example, with different ideas about how information should be organized, what topics are allowable, how stretches of talk like narratives should be structured, how shifts in topic should be signaled, and how to display things like respect and empathy. These different expectations are often manifested in subtle signals like word choice, pauses, rhythm and intonation, gaze, gestures and other non-verbal behavior which Gumperz (1982) calls 'contextualization cues'. This is why difficulties in such interactions are sometimes not a matter of explicit misunderstandings, but rather a more elusive sense of 'trouble' (Schegloff, 1987), a feeling that the interaction did not progress as smoothly or successfully as it might have. Because of this, such difficulties in 'intercultural communication' are often difficult to pinpoint and repair.

Erickson and Rittenberg (1987), for instance, have examined the difficulties Vietnamese and Polish physicians in the United States have in managing topics in their consultations. Topic management, they argue, requires two kinds of socio-cultural knowledge: an overall understanding of who has the right to talk about certain things at certain times, and a more specific understanding of how to manage the moment-by-moment conduct of interactions, for example how to show appropriate 'listenership' and how to draw proper inferences from utterances and other communicative behaviors. The problem with both of these kinds of knowledge is that they are rarely made explicit, and when things go wrong, people seldom point them out directly (Gumperz, 1982).

One area where difficulties often arise in health-related communication is in expectations about how information ought to be ordered. In a study in Britain, Roberts and her colleagues (2004) found that when explaining the reasons for their visits to doctors most speakers of British varieties of English followed a consistent format of beginning with a brief, context-setting introduction and moving on to a description of their symptoms. Speakers of other varieties of English, however, often diverged considerably from this structure, sometimes leaving off the context-setting, and sometimes spending so long setting the context that the doctor began to wonder what the main point of the visit was. Such variations in rhetorical strategies might result in doctors interrupting patients before they are able to fully express what is wrong with them, or in misinterpreting what is wrong with them due to lack of sufficient contextual information.

One particularly dramatic example of a mismatch of expectations about how information should be exchanged and topics should be managed in medical interviews is Scollon and Scollon's (1981, 2004) study of interactions between Athabaskan patients and non-Athabaskan doctors in Alaska, in which they found that doctors often complained that Athabaskan patients were uncooperative and Athabaskan patients complained that doctors never listened – they just asked endless questions. The problem, the Scollons argue, lies in the fact that for the Athabaskan patients, questions had an altogether different social function than they did for the doctors. For them, the main function of questions, especially when they come from authority figures, is not to get an answer, but to get the listener to think deeply about his or her improper behavior. In other words, questions function more like reprimands. At the same time, these patients believed that doctors should be able to infer what is wrong with them from direct observation and from listening to them talk about their daily affairs. To speak directly about their problems would be, in effect, pre-empting the doctor's opportunity to make his or her own inferences and would be seen as disrespectful. Typically, then, patients would approach consultations by offering stories about hunting trips or visiting relatives, which often seemed irrelevant to the doctors, who proceeded to try to turn the conversation to medical issues by asking direct questions about symptoms or health-related behavior. In response to these questions, the patients would do what they thought they were supposed to do: think deeply about their behavior and cultivate a sense of regret. In the end, the patients ended up leaving the consultations feeling that the doctors had spent a lot of time scolding them without really listening to try to find out what was wrong.

Sometimes intercultural misunderstandings can result from broader differences in expectations about power and interactional roles. This has been particularly evident as 'patient-centered' approaches to medical communication that have been developed in Europe and North America in the past two decades are exported to contexts where participants expect more 'doctor-centered' approaches. Smith (1999), for example, found that many of the patients he surveyed in Hong Kong were resistant to physicians who attempted to implement patient-centered communicative strategies, preferring doctors who would tell them what to do. The communicative behaviors they most valued in doctors were explanation- and advice-giving rather than listening and showing empathy. In some cultural contexts, writes Roberts (2010, p. 209), '"patient-centered" models … and the idea that more talk is likely to mean less misunderstanding … often do not work and even cause more confusion when talk itself is the problem.' Conversely, Erickson and Rittenberg (1987) found that foreign doctors in the US sometimes have difficulty adapting to patients who expect to take a more active role in medical interactions. Such observations highlight the dangers of making blanket generalizations about 'effective communication' across cultural contexts.

There are, however, as I mentioned above, dangers associated with focusing on 'cultural differences' when analyzing professional interaction around health and risk. One danger is assuming that differences exist a priori, independent of the way they are constructed moment-by-moment at sites of engagement. Just because a patient and physician have different native languages or come from different places does not necessarily mean that their encounter will be 'intercultural'. 'Differences and similarities', as Roberts and her colleagues (2005, p. 466) remind us, 'arise out of the encounter as it happens … Patients and GPs either "talk themselves into an intercultural encounter" or interculturality is simply not attended to.'

Another danger is that a focus on 'cultural' differences can lead analysts to ignore similarities, which might be even more relevant to the interaction. In their study of non-native English-speaking nurses working in a US psychiatric hospital, for example, Cameron and Williams (1997) found that even when language proficiency and cultural expectations about discourse presented barriers to communication, healthcare workers from different cultural backgrounds were, more often than not, able to work together successfully because of their skills at making inferences based on shared professional knowledge.

This last example illustrates a third danger, that of taking too narrow a view of 'culture' as having to do only with race, ethnicity, native language, or national origin. People, in fact, belong to a whole range of different kinds of 'cultures' connected to things like their professions and the institutions they work for (Cook-Gumperz and Messerman, 1999; Iedema and Scheeres, 2003), their gender (Fisher, 1995; West, 1984), their age (N. Coupland et al., 1991), and their social class (Todd, 1984). Even different kinds of physicians and different kinds of patients might 'bring along' different expectations about social practices and social identities to their interactions. In chapter 2, for example, I discussed a study which showed that HIV specialist doctors and nurses in Hong Kong were concerned about their patients' reluctance to talk about non-medical, 'lifeworld' topics, while their HIV-positive patients preferred to limit what they discussed in medical encounters to topics like symptoms and medications. The patients in this example may have been particularly reticent not because they were 'Chinese', but because they were certain kinds of patients for whom disclosure of personal information might have been seen as particularly problematic, and the doctors and nurses may have been unusually communicative because they belonged to a special 'culture' of HIV specialist healthcare workers who had been steeped in literature about the psycho-social dimensions of AIDS and the importance of communicating with their patients.

The fact is, we are all members of multiple, overlapping and intersecting cultures or 'discourse systems' (Scollon et al., 2012). Patients and doctors are, at the same time, men and women, gays and straights, Christians and Buddhists. Not all of these identities, of course, are relevant to the medical encounter, but they exist as resources which participants draw on as they negotiate professional encounters. In fact, no matter who we are talking to, whether it be our doctor, our parents or our spouse, we might find that we have 'brought along' a range of different practices and identities from the multiple discourse systems in which we participate, and we need to choose which to appropriate at any given moment. A sometimes more vexing issue, then, when it comes to intercultural communication, is not the intercultural communication which occurs *between* people but that which occurs *within* them as they struggle to reconcile the sometimes conflicting expectations about 'what they are doing' and 'who they are being' that they bring to interactions. The teenagers discussed by Eggert and Nicholas (1992) (see chapter 5), for example, who skip school and take drugs but still maintain high grade point averages, need to carefully manage different 'cultural identities' (as, for example, 'skippers', 'jocks', and 'geeks') as they navigate the school day.

Often, however, in communication about health and risk, the notion of 'culture' itself is 'technologized', becoming a tool that is appropriated by people in order to take certain actions or claim and impute certain identities. People might, for example, invoke their own 'culture' as a reason for engaging in a particular kind of health-related behavior or as a justification for feelings of immunity from certain health hazards, or may use the 'culture' of other groups as an explanation for their vulnerability to certain diseases. In the late 1990s I attended a seminar on 'AIDS Prevention in Chinese Communities' where a representative from Taiwan was rebuked by a representative from Hong Kong for the sexually explicit prevention materials for gay men he had designed. 'We could never use such materials in Hong Kong,' she said, 'because we're Chinese and so don't like to talk so openly about sex', apparently forgetting that the man she was addressing was also 'Chinese'.

Professional and institutional discourse systems

To say that healthcare is becoming an increasingly multicultural enterprise does not just mean that it involves more and more patients and healthcare workers from different countries interacting, but also that it increasingly involves healthcare workers from different professional groups working together. Hospitals and clinics are complex networks of knowledge and competence distributed across different departments and professions (Måseide, 2007a). While all employees of the hospital might be seen to share interpretative practices by virtue of their common participation in an institutional or 'corporate' discourse system (Scollon et al., 2012), they also hold different kinds of knowledge and skills, engage in different kinds of interactions, and use different forms of discourse based on the professional discourse systems in which they participate. Iedema and his colleagues (2006, p. 1126) argue that healthcare is increasingly characterized by what they call 'interactive volatility', a phenomenon in which people with different ways of discursively constructing knowledge and communicating about it must work together to negotiate meaning.

Encounters between professionals in different fields can be challenging for a number of reasons. The most obvious has to do with the different kinds of 'professional vision' (Goodwin, 1994) they might bring to a case and the different propositions they might subscribe to regarding diagnosis and treatment. Peräkylä and her colleagues (2005) broadly refer to these as 'treatment theories'. Different professional discourse systems, they point out, also have different notions about the way information about health should be *communicated*, with whom it should be shared, and the interactional roles and responsibilities of different people in health-related interactions. Peräkylä and her colleagues refer to these as the 'interaction theories'. When working in interdisciplinary teams, healthcare workers are faced with the task of making themselves accountable for both of these kinds of theories.

Key questions for those studying professional communication in medicine, then, are how individuals from different professions manage to interact successfully, and in what ways institutions facilitate these interactions, without compromising professional autonomy and identity. These questions touch on two of the concepts I discussed earlier in this book, the first being the prevalence of *interdiscursivity* in communication about health and risk, and the challenges and opportunities that arise when different, sometimes competing 'voices' interact in texts and at sites of engagement, and the second being the *organizing* power of discourse itself – the ways texts and talk shape interactions and social relationships.

Just as new sets of professional practices and professional relationships have developed in healthcare institutions to facilitate the work of interdisciplinary care teams, new kinds of texts and discourse practices have also been developed to support and sustain these practices and relationships, texts and practices like treatment guidelines, benchmarks, incident reporting, 'adverse event' investigations, patient complaint procedures, and resource utilization audits (Iedema et al., 2005).

The primary process developed in post-bureaucratic organizations to deal with increased interdiscursivity is what Iedema and Scheeres (2003) call *talking work*. The modern hospital, like the modern corporation, works to create and sustain institutional orders through engaging workers in various exercises of *joint entextualization* in which they both reflect upon and make themselves accountable for their performance. One example of this in hospital settings is the joint creation of clinical artifacts such as X-rays and laboratory tests. In chapter 6 I discussed how such technologies can sometimes result in the fragmentation of the patient's body as it is dispersed across different institutional units and zones of expertise. At the same time, such artifacts can also serve to facilitate institutional cohesion, constructing intertextual links across units and professions. Måseide (2007b), for example, talks about how the artifact of the X-ray is collaboratively produced through multi-professional collaboration, beginning with the written request for an X-ray from the physician, which creates the framework for the medical problem under investigation, progressing through discussions between the physician and radiologist about the aspects of the image that are clinically relevant, and culminating with the radiologist's written report and the physician's diagnosis based on it.

Another such act of joint entextualization which I discussed in the last chapter is the electronic medical record. Iedema (2003b) argues that medical records serve as important 'organizing discourses' for hospitals and clinics by transforming the specific and immediate circumstances of the individual patient into standard, generalizable artifacts that function as 'boundary objects' (Star and Greisemer, 1989), mediating among professionals, departments, and institutions. Despite the drawbacks of electronic medical records that I pointed out in the last chapter, the standardization imposed by them does facilitate communication between different caregivers and different departments and allows data from one patient to be easily compared or aggregated with data from other patients for research and administrative purposes. 'Only as clinical notation disconnects from the here-and-now in this way,' writes Iedema (2003b, p. 69), 'is its discourse able to create "lines of force" across time, space, and agency. Only then does its discourse "organize"' (see also Star and Greisemer, 1989; Reddy et al., 2001).

Apart from medical records, interdisciplinary teams engage in other kinds of joint entextualization in which they are made discursively accountable to one another. Iedema and Scheeres (2003, p. 326), for instance, analyze the ways teams produce 'multidisciplinary clinical pathways', forms of discourse in which the tasks and responsibilities of different members of the team are laid out and 'explicitly linked to resource requirements, clinical benchmarks, [and] quality assurance measures' (p. 326). Such texts compel members to articulate their work within a common set of discursive constraints. Iedema and Scheeres argue that such practices can be both disruptive and empowering: disruptive because they compel people to 'rewrite' not just their practices, but also their professional identities, and empowering because they create opportunities for individuals to simultaneously reflect on intra-professional practices and come to an understanding of how these practices fit into the bigger picture of the institution. Explaining what you do to people who do not share the same assumptions you do can encourage a kind of reflexivity about one's work which, like the reflexivity resulting from the activities of self-entextualization I discussed in the last chapter, sets up feedback loops that facilitate continual improvement. At the same time, while team members make themselves accountable to one another, they also participate in co-managing the accountability of the team as a whole, which encourages them to see themselves as contributing to more universal, institutional discourse.

There are, of course, downsides to such 'organizing discourses'. Rather than facilitating trust and communication, they might foster suspicion and cynicism, and rather than fostering innovation, they might instead foster bureaucratic rigidity. When such discourses are imposed from the top down, as they often are, they can actually interfere with the 'organic' development of processes of shared decision-making (G. P. Martin and Finn, 2011). Bokhour (2006), in her analysis of the ways teams in hospitals work together to write 'interdisciplinary treatment plans', notes how often the writing of the plan to fulfill the bureaucratic requirements of the institution comes to be seen as the primary aim of team meetings, sometimes detracting from more useful discussions about patient needs. In fact, more than 25 percent of utterances she recorded at such meetings dealt exclusively with how things should be 'worded' on the reporting form. As team members focus on fulfilling institutional goals, Bokhour observes, 'crucial social and personal information about patients is often excluded' (p. 359). When asked about the main purpose of meetings, one team member who participated in the study said, 'It's all about the paper' (p. 255). Cook-Gumperz and Messerman (1999) make similar observations in their analysis of team meetings, noting that consensus among disparate professionals is often 'manufactured' by backgrounding professional concerns and focusing on the institutionally appropriate language that is to be used in writing the patient's care plan.

On a broader level, tension between professional and institutional discourse systems might arise as professionals act to retain their control over specialized knowledge through their unique forms of discourse, and institutions strive to routinize such knowledge through standardized forms of 'organizing discourse'. Crawford and his colleagues (2008), for example, examine the disjunction between the clinical practices of doctors and nurses in an acute psychiatric care unit and the ideals of clinical governance stipulated by hospital administrators, and scholars of medical interpreting (see for example Angelelli, 2012; Davidson, 2000) have noted how the local knowledge and practices interpreters develop to deal with specific clinical contexts often contradict both institutional expectations about how they should behave and what the 'codes of ethics' of professional associations prescribe.

Health, risk, and 'communities'

Another common way of thinking about the effect of group affiliation on health and risk is in terms of 'communities'. The notion of 'community' began to gain currency in the field of health promotion in the 1960s, following the insights gained from early epidemiological studies of disease risk like the groundbreaking Framingham Heart Study (Kannel et al., 1962). While the earliest prevention programs to come out of these studies focused on the identification and treatment of 'high-risk individuals', by the 1970s programs like the Stanford Three-Community Study (Blackburn, 1983) began to target 'high-risk groups'. In the 1980s, however, partly as a result of the stigmatization of certain segments of the population in the early days of the AIDS epidemic, the epidemiological concept of 'risk group' began to fall out of favor, criticized by researchers, activists, and social commentators as both discriminatory and reductionist (see for example Treichler, 1988b). The category of 'risk group', it was argued, not only fails to capture the complex and dynamic nature of group affiliation in social life, but actually has the potential to *undermine* health promotion efforts by giving the impression that risk is a matter of *who* people are rather than *what* they do or the social circumstances in which they live (Clatts, 1995). By the 1990s, in most public health circles in the industrialized world the term 'risk group' had been replaced with the term 'vulnerable community'.

This terminological evolution illustrates the fact that the label we attach to a social group – whether we call it a 'culture', a 'community', or a 'risk group' – serves to make certain aspects of it and its members criterial. The term 'risk group' makes criterial the notion of *risk* and assigns agency for this risk to members of the group. Moreover, the word 'group' suggests nothing else that binds these people together beyond 'risk'. The term 'vulnerable community', on the other hand, constructs individuals whose risk for developing a particular disease or condition is less a matter of their own intentional actions and more a matter of outside forces and social conditions (such as poverty, discrimination, and inadequate education). Furthermore, the word 'community' suggests a more organic, naturally occurring entity whose existence is not dependent on vulnerability.

In community-based health promotion, communities themselves are seen as mechanisms for behavior change. Rather than staging top-down 'interventions' from the outside, community-based health promoters attempt to tap into indigenous processes of communication and socialization within communities, wherever possible involving community members as 'peer educators' and 'role models' (Clements and Buczkiewicz, 1993; Perry and Sieving, 1993). The reasoning behind this approach rests on the assumption that individuals' perceptions of health and risk develop through their interaction with peers (Douglas and Calvez, 1990), and that often people trust peers more than they do experts (Perry, 1989; Topol, 2012).

Perhaps the most famous example of successful community-based health promotion is the response of gay communities in North America, Europe, and Australia to AIDS in the early 1980s at a time when the governments of these countries were still a long way from making it a public health priority (King, 1993; Kippax et al., 1993; Watney, 1990). In fact, it was the groundbreaking pamphlet 'How to Have Sex in an Epidemic' (Berkowitz and Callen, 1983), published by members of the gay community in New York before the cause of AIDS had even been discovered, in which the approach to HIV prevention that dominates public health today was first articulated. The early success within these communities of fostering behavior change, argues Watney (1990), came from promoting 'safer sex' not as a series of techniques to be mastered by individuals but a constellation of collective cultural practices through which people could claim and impute certain social identities. The AIDS epidemic, in fact, was a major impetus for the health promotion establishment in the 1990s to embrace community-based approaches to a wide range of public health issues (Rhodes, 1994).

With the exception of HIV prevention, however, the evidence from more than four decades of community-based health promotion shows that it has had only a modest impact on changing people's behavior or improving their health (Merzel and D'Afflitti, 2003). Community-based programs have had disappointing results in, for example, getting people to eat better (Dunt, Day, and Pirkis, 2007), getting them to stop smoking (Schofield et al., 1991), and getting heterosexuals to use condoms with casual sexual partners (Ng et al., 2011). There have even been studies that question the most central theoretical assumption of the approach: the extent to which people actually do influence the health behavior of their peers (Mitchell and West, 1996). Do people adopt the behaviors of people in the communities in which they participate, critics ask, or do they participate in these communities because the people in them engage in behaviors similar to theirs?

The biggest problem in understanding why some community-based approaches to health and risk seem to work while others do not lies in the fact that, just as with the word 'culture', when people use the word 'community' in relation to health and risk, they often mean different things at different times. McLeroy and his colleagues (2003), in their review of community-based interventions, note considerable variation in the ways different programs define 'community', some seeing community as a *setting* in which health promotion takes place, some seeing it as a *group of people targeted* for certain messages, some seeing it as a *resource* for assisting health promoters in delivering messages, and some seeing it as an *agent* in designing and delivering the intervention. It is fair to assume that there must also be considerable variation among the groups at the receiving end of these programs. Do these people actually see themselves as 'communities', and if so, what are the social and discursive processes which hold them together and determine who is a member and who is not?

An applied linguistic view of community begins with the relationship between discourse and action with which I began this book. Whenever people take social actions, they do so by drawing on shared resources or 'cultural tools' and adapting them to their particular goals and circumstances. Every time they do so they reproduce certain social practices and claim membership in the social groups associated with these practices (Norris and Jones, 2005; Scollon, 2001b). A gay man who uses a condom when having sex, a mother who only buys organic vegetables for her family, and a man who records his daily exercise using Nike+ are reproducing the practices of 'safe sex', 'healthy eating', and 'regular exercise', and also reproducing themselves as certain kinds of people.

Of course it takes more than just shared social practices to create a community. Just because I buy organic food doesn't necessarily make me part of a 'community of healthy eaters' and just because I exercise regularly doesn't make me a member of a 'community of exercisers'. There must be a process by which this combination of shared social practices and shared social identities over time come to be regarded by the people engaged in them as a recognizable entity. In other words, communities themselves must be *technologized* or 'talked into existence' by their members through the day-to-day production and consumption of texts and the day-to-day engagement in social interactions.

Imagined communities and imaginary protections

Wertsch (2001) sees the social construction of communities in terms of three 'stages' of technologization. The first stage is commensurate with what Lave and Wenger (1991) call 'communities of practice', groups of people who 'do things together'. Examples of such communities might be gay men who congregate at a certain public sex venue, the 'skippers' in Eggert and Nicholas' (1992) research who skip class together and 'get high', and amateur athletes who meet up regularly to train for a triathlon. In many ways, the notion of 'communities of practice' is extremely circumscribed, defined in terms of mutual engagement and shared goals. Men who cruise for sex in public parks in China and in 'beats' in Sydney are not members of the same 'community of practice', nor are teenagers who skip school in San Diego in the same community of practice as those who skip school in London. While the practices these groups engage in may be similar, they are not the same. In communities of practice, practices are always local, always defined by the concrete group of people who perform them at specific places and times.

The narrowness of this definition, however, does not make it less useful when it comes to understanding health and risk. Some, in fact, might argue that this narrow, concrete focus on practice is the best place to start when considering how to understand and change people's health behavior. The most important contribution this perspective makes is the shift of focus it offers away from the individualistic theories of learning and behavior change I discussed in chapter 5, which reduce us to blaming individuals for their 'poor health choices', to a theory of learning and behavior change that sees it as a matter of participation in a social group.

At the same time, this narrow view of community limits our understanding of how social practices and social identities related to health and risk come to transcend particular geographically defined groups to be taken up by people who do not 'do things together', but who essentially 'do the same things'. Wertsch calls these 'implicit communities' – communities that are based not on shared actions, but on shared tools and practices that transcend space and time. In this second stage of technologization, these shared tools and practices provide the *potential* for groups of people who have never met one another to grow into 'symbolic' communities by creating representations of themselves around these tools and practices.

The final stage in the technologization of communities is what Wertsch (2001), after Benedict Anderson (1991), calls 'imagined communities', communities which have, to varying degrees, come to be recognized as such by members. In 'imagined communities', says Wertsch (2001, p. 3) 'there is an emphasis given to recognizing or imagining the collectivity and to creating or reproducing it.'

For Wertsch, as for Anderson, the primary process through which communities come to 'imagine themselves' is the production and consumption of *texts*. For Anderson (1991) the prototypical *imagined community* – the nation-state – was made possible by the invention of the printing press, which allowed for textual representations of certain kinds of people, certain kinds of social practices, and the *idea* of 'the country' to be widely circulated. Similarly, the mass media and internet today have played a major role in the imagination of countless communities, from the 'barebacker community' (Shernoff, 2006), which traffics in erotic stories of unsafe sex, to the 'autism community' (Mnookin, 2011), which traffics in stories about how members believe their children developed autism and what they are doing about it (see chapter 3). What separates imagined communities from implicit communities is that members can use their membership itself (or 'emblems' of that membership like biohazard tattoos) to take social actions.

Imagined communities have an important effect on health and risk behavior because they allow for certain social practices and social identities to spread across time and space. The texts, discursive practices, and channels of communication that hold communities together can also serve to disseminate innovations such as 'safer sex'. In this regard, it might be argued that the reason community-based HIV prevention was more effective in the 1980s among gay men (as opposed, for example, to IV drug users) was because the 'gay community' had already developed a strong 'discursive infrastructure' for imagining itself as a community, including a range of common texts, symbols, practices, and identities. Of course, the discursive infrastructures of imagined communities can also facilitate the spread of 'unhealthy' or 'risky' behaviors, making it possible, for example, for social practices like 'barebacking' to be quickly technologized and spread throughout the community.

Not surprisingly, helping to build 'strong communities' through facilitating these processes of 'imagining' has been seen by some as the ultimate goal of community-based health promotion (Minkler, 1997). Strong communities, it is argued, create channels through which information about healthy behaviors can be spread and act as support systems for sustaining that behavior. At the same time, strong communities can also act as obstacles to healthy behaviors. One way they do this can be seen in the example of attitudes towards HIV risk among different groups with which I began this chapter. The imagining of my group (be it gays or straights, 'zegoch' or 'comrades') as 'safe' and the invention of other groups (be they gays or straights, drug addicts or prostitutes) as 'risky' helps to create in communities what Mendés-Leite (1998) calls 'imaginary protections', beliefs that community affiliation itself constitutes protection against health risks.

Mendés-Leite emphasizes that what distinguishes imaginary protections is not their 'irrationality' but their 'rationality'. They are strategies groups use to rationalize behaviors they do not wish to give up. 'Imaginary protections', however, do more than just relieve cognitive dissonance. They can also serve as important tools for the imagination of community itself. In my study of the rise of the gay community in China in the 1990s (Jones, 2002a, 2007), for example, I found that the strategy of downplaying their vulnerability to HIV functioned as a way for members of the nascent gay community to claim 'cultural citizenship' in a discursive environment in which homosexuals had previously been constructed as hooligans, counter-revolutionaries, and carriers of disease. By claiming invulnerability to AIDS, gay men were able to draw boundaries between themselves and groups like 'migrant workers', 'prostitutes', and 'drug addicts'. The consequence of these 'imaginary protections' was, of course, *greater* vulnerability to HIV, since practices like using condoms were seen to compromise the imagined identity these men had cultivated for themselves. The point of this example is that the discursive processes used to construct 'imaginary protections' are sometimes also central to the imagination of community in the first place. The 'imaginary protections' that made the men I studied in China more vulnerable to HIV were at the same time tools they used to open up spaces for community-empowerment and to claim social legitimacy.

What are the implications of this discussion for health and risk communication and 'community-based' health promotion? First, it highlights the fact that those who wish to study communities or design health-promotion programs for them must differentiate between the ways they have 'invented' these communities in their own minds and the ways community members actually imagine themselves. Second, we must aspire to understand the dynamic and contingent discursive processes through which communities are constructed and sustained. Finally, we must seek to understand how communities exist not just in the minds of their members but also in their *actions*, how particular social practices (like 'safer sex' or 'barebacking') themselves become ways of belonging to a community.

Social networks: 'going viral'

More recently scholars of health and risk have turned their attention to social structures that are not characterized by common practices, common goals, or common processes of 'imagining', but rather by the sometimes tenuous social ties that link people with others in webs of relationships known as *social networks*. Social networks include people whom we know well and with whom we interact regularly, as well as people we hardly know at all who may belong to different 'communities' or different 'cultures'. The analysis of social networks focuses on how the patterns of relationships between people, rather than characteristics or beliefs of the people themselves, serve to enable or constrain social actions.

What is important about social networks from the point of view of health and risk is that research has shown that even in the absence of frequent social contact, shared practices and shared processes of 'imagining', health beliefs, and behaviors (as well as pathogens like germs and viruses) spread through social networks with remarkable efficiency. If people in your social network are obese, you are more likely to be obese, and if people in your social network smoke, you are more likely to smoke, whether or not you interact with these people (Christakis and Fowler, 2007, 2008).

The roots of social network theory can be traced back to the sociologists Emile Durkheim and George Simmel. Durkheim, in his classic work on suicide (1952, first published in 1897), demonstrated how individual pathology can be seen as a function of social connectedness. Among other things, he found that the rate of suicide in Europe was higher among Protestants than among Catholics or Jews, not, he surmised, because of differences in beliefs, but because of differences in the strength of social ties. Two decades later, George Simmel put forth a detailed theory of 'social geometry', showing how social relationships are affected by patterns of social organization (Simmel, 1955, first published in 1922). The term 'social net-work', however, was not used until the 1950s when it was developed to analyze the ways social ties that cut across traditional groups like family, community, and class affect things like economic standing and political activity (Barnes, 1954; Bott, 1957). The concept was first used in the field of public health in the 1970s when a series of studies appeared showing rates of mortality from almost any cause of death can be predicted by analyzing social ties (Cassel, 1976; Cobb, 1976). Nowadays, social network analysis is a staple methodology of social epidemiology, providing insights into how social ties serve as vectors for the spread of infectious diseases as well as the dispersion of health and risk behaviors (see for example Laumann et al., 1989). As Christakis and Fowler (2007, p. 379) put it, 'people are connected, and so their health is connected.'

With the development of the internet and Web 2.0 technologies, there has been increased interest in the effect of online social networks on health and risk. Online social networks like Facebook function partly as a way to make already existent offline social networks more explicit. The ethos of online social networks, which encourages the frequent sharing of personal information (see chapter 7), serves to make members of the network and what they do more visible to other members, facilitating the diffusion of information, behavior, and attitudes.

It is perhaps fitting that the most prevalent metaphors for the rapid spread of ideas through social networks are from medicine. The evolutionary biologist Richard Dawkins, for example, compares what he calls *memes*, ideas that spread rapidly through social networks, to both genes and viruses. He writes,

> Just as genes propagate themselves in the gene pool by leaping from body to body via sperms or eggs, so memes propagate themselves in the meme pool by leaping from brain to brain via a process which, in the broad sense, can be called imitation. ... When you plant a fertile meme in my mind you literally parasitize my brain, turning it into a vehicle for the meme's propagation in just the way that a virus may parasitize the genetic mechanism of a host cell.
>
> (Dawkins, 2006, p. 192)

In popular parlance, when we speak of ideas, behaviors, and cultural products that have disseminated quickly through online social networks we frequently describe them as having 'gone viral'.

One example of this occurred in 2009 when news of an experimental treatment for MS touted by surgeon Paolo Zamboni, which involved inflating a tiny balloon inside twisted veins in the patient's neck, spread quickly through online social networks like YouTube and Facebook, creating such a demand for the therapy that a number of hospitals and private practices began offering it, despite the fact that there was no conclusive evidence of either its safety or its effectiveness (Moisse, 2011). Some celebrated this phenomenon as evidence of the potential of online social networks to foster patient empowerment (Chafe et al., 2011). Others, however, warned of the dangers involved in hyping unproven procedures (Butler, 2012). In 2012 the U.S. Food and Drug Administration issued a warning linking the therapy to patient injuries and deaths (U.S. Food and Drug Administration, 2012). Nevertheless, demands from patients for greater access to the treatment and increased research funding to prove its effectiveness have continued unabated, fuelled by social media.

The internet can also function as a tool for *expanding* social networks and *creating* new ones. This potential is particularly evident in the growth of online sexual networks, especially among gay men, making use of such sites as Gaydar.com, Manhunt.com, and, more recently, mobile, GPS-powered applications such as Grindr to find sexual partners (Gudelunas, 2012; Jones, 2005b, 2012). The tools available on such sites for screening profiles based on things like body type and sexual preferences, and for easily initiating relationships, make them an efficient means for disseminating and amplifying various types of sexual behavior and values as well as sexually transmitted infections (Halkitis and Parsons, 2003).

The internet has also made possible the formation of networks of people who share information about their health. Unlike more traditional 'online support groups' (Hamilton, 1998; Stommel, 2009), which operate more like 'communities' in which people coalesce around common interests or goals, 'health social networks' such as PatientsLikeMe, CureTogether, and 23andMe (see chapter 7) are looser structures in which people with a wide range of health conditions, motivations, and interests exchange information which can be aggregated and used to help individuals make better health decisions. Such networks are distinguished by their porous boundaries, low barriers to entry, and the tools they provide for the collection and aggregation of information from participants. While sometimes participants in such networks interact in online forums or discussion groups, these networks do not depend on individuals engaging directly with one another at all or aligning to any common values or goals (Frost and Massagli, 2008; Haythornthwaite, 2009).

Perhaps the best example of this sort of 'health social network' is the website PatientsLikeMe, established in 2004 by the brothers of a patient with amyotrophic lateral sclerosis (ALS) to help him exchange experiences with other patients. Currently the site has over 50,000 members with a wide variety of diseases and medical conditions, who interact using a combination of social networking tools like those found on Facebook and information-recording tools like those found in electronic personal health record systems. Users of the site have access to the personal health information of all the other users (including their symptoms, the treatments they have undergone, the progression of their diseases or conditions, and the lifestyles they lead).

As with sites like 23andMe, however, 'health social networks' raise important questions about patient privacy and the commodification of personal health information. As the PatientsLikeMe website explains to users, 'We take the information patients like you share about your experience with the disease and sell it to our partners (i.e. companies that are developing or selling products to patients). These products may include drugs, devices, equipment, insurance, and medical services.' While it can be argued that by selling aggregated data from users, operators of health social networks contribute to advancements in medical knowledge that eventually benefit patients, it might also be argued that in gathering and selling the information patients 'share' with *each other*, companies 'blur the boundaries of coercion and consent' (Vicdan and Dholakia, 2013, p. 6). As Brubaker and his colleagues (2010) argue, by mixing discourses of 'transparency' and 'collaboration' in patient–patient interactions with the corporate interests of the company, operators of health social networks gloss over important questions regarding patients' rights to control what is done with their health information.

The 'organizing discourses' of social networks

As with 'cultures' and 'communities', the key questions we must ask about social networks are, first, how they form and, second, how they work to influence people's actions around health and risk. Most work on social networks has focused on examining patterns of social ties, analyzing their 'strength' or 'weakness', observing the flows of social and material resources through them, and representing this information in the form of relational matrices and sociograms. From the point of view of applied linguistics, however, it is difficult to talk about social ties of any kind without considering how those ties are *discursively* constituted, and difficult to discuss 'flows' of resources without taking into account the 'itineraries' along which discourse travels as it is entextualized, decontextualized, and recontextualized in various sites of engagement (see chapter 2).

Some social network analysts have recognized the discursive basis of social networks, most famously Dunbar (1996), who argues that language itself evolved as a means to sustain network ties. Seemingly trivial speech genres like gossip, he argues, have important functions in human societies, providing an efficient way for people to build and maintain social networks and regulate flows of resources through them. Similarly, Mische and White (1998) insist that network relations and discursive processes are co-constitutive – discourse produces networks and networks produce discourse. The chief forms of discourse they see as driving the formation and maintenance of social networks are what they call 'conversations' and 'stories'. By 'conversations' they mean something like what Dunbar broadly defines as 'gossip', 'free flowing discursive exchanges that help to smooth relational mixing' (p. 696). By 'stories' they mean something like what I have been calling 'storylines', expectations about how certain kinds of social exchanges ought to unfold based on shared sets of 'technologized' social practices and social identities.

Understanding the ways everyday conversations and shared storylines facilitate the maintenance of social networks and the flows of social practices and social identities through them introduces considerable methodological challenges for applied linguists. Traditional methods of text and conversation analysis and even ethnographic tools like participant observation are often not suited to studying the complex pathways along which discourse travels in social networks or to capturing the sometimes subtle ways meanings change as they travel along these pathways.

One attempt to address these difficulties which is also relevant to the study of health and risk communication is Watkins, Swindler and Biruk's (2008) use of what they call 'hearsay ethnography' to study how information and attitudes about AIDS spreads through social networks in villages in rural Malawi. Using a method in which paid informants kept diaries in which they recorded overheard conversations related to HIV/AIDS throughout their day, Watkins and her colleagues are able to show the role of both 'conversations' and 'storylines' in the dissemination of health information and practices across traditional social boundaries of kinship, gender, age, social status, and tribe. What they found is that health beliefs and behaviors are spread not so much through formal educational discourse, but rather through everyday relational discourse as people gossip, entertain one another, seek advice and pursue various personal agendas in a range of quotidian contexts. As people share news about friends, friends of friends, and more distantly removed acquaintances, their health, sexual behavior, family problems and other aspects of their lives, they pull together bits and pieces of knowledge distributed throughout the network, gradually formulating 'storylines' about AIDS, how it is spread and what can be done to prevent it that are released back into the network to spread into other contexts where they function as 'heuristics' (Abelson, 1976) for other conversations and for actions around things like sex.

In chapters 4 and 5 I considered situated interactions around health and risk in various sites of engagement, including both professional and non-professional contexts. My discussion, however, was chiefly limited to the analysis of focused, dyadic interactions and did not concentrate so much on how interactions at multiple sites of engagement are linked together. Work like that of Watkins and her colleagues reminds us of the danger of trying to study social interactions in isolation, as if the only relevant 'participants' are those that are physically co-present. Many analytical methods in the social sciences, Watkins and her colleagues argue, evoke the image of interaction

> as something like a ping-pong game in which one player hits the ball to another who responds in turn. … Rather than a game of ping-pong, hearsay ethnography's social space is more like a game of pool, with multiple players and multiple balls going this way and that.
>
> *(Watkins et al., 2008, p. 29).*

The discursive characteristics of online social networks that distinguish them from the kinds of social networks examined by Watkins and her colleagues are the ways they *lower the social costs* of engaging in 'conversations', the way they provide *templates* for the standardization of social identities and storylines, the way they facilitate the *filtering* of information as it flows through the network, and the *persistence* of conversations within the network which both functions to strengthen network ties and provides opportunities for researchers to more easily trace the flows of discourse through these networks.

One of the most important changes digital tools have brought to the way we communicate is to lower the barriers to engaging in what Malinowski (1923) calls *phatic* communication, communication whose main purpose is to strengthen human relationships and provide social support rather than to exchange information (Jones and Hafner, 2012). Text messaging and microblogging tools make it possible for people to engage in the kind of 'conversations' Watkins and her colleagues examine from a distance, and to broadcast their health and risk-related behavior to others on a regular basis (through, for example, status updates about going to the gym or eating certain kinds of food). These tools also make it more convenient for people to turn to their social networks rather than professionals for advice on health and risk, and to form 'feedback loops' with people who reinforce their health and risk-taking behaviors. Teenagers with eating disorders, for example, join online networks of like-minded people like 'Starving for Perfection' (proanaskinnyblog.blogspot.com), which provide for them a constant stream of positive reinforcement and advice about practices like self-induced vomiting, and users of Nike+ can adjust the settings on their iPhones so their progress as they run is broadcast to their Facebook page, and whenever a member of their social network 'likes' it, a 'cheer' is played through their headphones.

Another way digital media help to organize social networks is through creating standardized structures or 'templates' for people to share information about themselves, their behaviors, and their desires. One of the reasons online social networks are such an efficient way for gay men interested in 'barebacking' to find willing partners, for example, is that all members of such networks submit standardized 'profile information', which makes things like preferences about condom use easily searchable. Such profiles help to technologize social identities and social practices within these networks by making certain kinds of information about users criterial and other kinds of information irrelevant. Similarly, PatientsLikeMe asks users to provide information about their medical conditions, symptoms, and treatments in a standardized format that allows for little variation. In a way, then, many online social networks suffer the same drawbacks as electronic medical records, forcing people to fit themselves into sets of predetermined categories and discouraging alternative entextualizations. At the same time, as with electronic medical records, this is also what makes such sites such efficient 'organizing discourses' for social networks, allowing users' information to be easily decontextualized and aggregated with that of other users in ways that are beneficial both to users and to the companies to which this information is sold.

A third way online tools affect the way discourse circulates through social networks is through facilitating *social filtering* (Jones and Hafner, 2012). All social networks serve as 'social filters', amplifying certain information and certain representations of reality and filtering out others. This is one of the chief mechanisms by which social networks function to reinforce health-related values and behaviors. What the Malawian villagers in Watkins, Swindler and Biruk's studies know about HIV transmission and prevention is filtered through the cognitive frames, interests, and prejudices of various people as it passes through the social network. Similarly, news about health and risk that reaches us through online social networks is filtered based on the interests and goals of the users of these networks. Blogs like 'Starving for Perfection', for example, collect and amplify pro-anorexia information for users and filter out information on health dangers, and anti-vaccination websites amplify studies that point to the dangers of vaccinations and downplay those demonstrating their safety. Where online social networks differ dramatically from offline networks is that they make social filtering so much more efficient, sometimes even automating the process. Items that appear on users' newsfeeds in Facebook, for example, are chosen by an algorithm that sorts them based on users' past behavior. Even search engines function as filters for information: Google's algorithm, for example, returns results based on users' behavior in clicking on previous results. What this means for the dissemination of health and risk information is that, more often than not, because of the online social networks that they belong to and their own past browsing history, people will find information that reinforces their health beliefs and practices rather than challenges them. Those who believe that vaccinations cause autism are likely to be confirmed in that belief, and anorexic teenagers are likely to get the impression that their behavior is more widespread and accepted than it actually is.

Finally, digital tools help to maintain and strengthen social networks because the 'conversations' that hold these networks together are 'persistent'. They remain on servers, available for people to browse through weeks, months, and years after they occur. What this also means is that the 'conversations' that travel through online social networks are much more visible to analysts, making it easier to track how meanings change as they are negotiated across a range of strong and weak social ties. In a study I did on how gay men talk about sex and AIDS in online discussion forums (Jones, 2009b), I observed how attitudes and knowledge about AIDS are spread through sexual stories, rumors, gossip, and insults that circulate through free-wheeling 'polylogues' (Marcocia, 2004) of multiple intertwining interactions among multiple users. In my analysis of a thread called 'Not using condoms ... > <', for example, I explored how the confession of a user that he doesn't use condoms with his boyfriend resulted in multiple competing conversations through which users transformed the topics of AIDS and safe sex into tools for positioning themselves and others within the social network. Such complex conversational phenomena, I argued, serve to remind health promoters that the 'information' they give to people about health can undergo profound and sometimes unpredictable transformations as it is filtered through social networks in which members engage in complex and dynamic processes of trading, reinforcing, resisting, and reinterpreting social identities.

*

In this chapter I have examined how various social structures such as 'cultures', professional discourse systems, communities, and social networks affect how people communicate about health and risk. I have analyzed both how social groups organize discourse, and how discourse functions to organize social groups. Understanding the ways language and communication contribute to the formation and main-tenance of groups and to the socialization of members into different kinds of social practices and social identities, I have argued, is crucial for understanding health and risk behavior. At the same time, discourse about health and risk can also play an important role in promoting a sense of group identity and policing the boundaries that separate members from non-members.

In chapter 3 I discussed how different 'discourse communities' (such as scientists and laypeople) draw on different processes of entextualization to represent reality and manage their social relationships. My observations in this chapter of the dis-cursive dynamics within groups add to that discussion, demonstrating how these processes of entextualization can themselves function as 'organizing discourses', creating group cohesion or providing discursive bridges from one group to another. This is an important point when we consider how discourse about health and risk changes as it moves from group to group, and from person to person within groups, being strategically appropriated and adapted for different purposes. It is also important in light of the new forms of group dynamics made possible by digital media, which have changed the participation frameworks and the 'economies of knowledge' within which people take action around health and risk (Richardson, 2003; Topol, 2012).

9

CONCLUSION

Discourse itineraries and research itineraries

The genetic test I got with 23andMe was worth every penny of the $299 I spent on it. Since receiving my report, I've appropriated my 'entextualized genome' to perform a whole host of useful actions. As I mentioned in chapter 7, I used it to consult with my doctor about my risk of developing colon cancer and to schedule a colonoscopy. I also used it to get a referral to see an ophthalmologist since I carry a variant of the CHF gene which is associated with age-related macular degeneration, a condition my mother suffers from. I altered my running regimen to include more sprints after finding out that I carry the R allele of the ACTN3 gene associated with rapid muscle contractions. I even used the test to comfort myself after failing my driving test, noting that I carry a variant of rs6265 associated with impaired motor-skills learning. At least I have the A allele of that gene, which has also been found to be protective against depression when carriers are subjected to repeated defeat.

Where my genetic test has turned out to be the most useful, however, is in giving me something to talk about at social gatherings. Whenever there is an uncomfortable lull in the conversation at a dinner party, all I have to do is bring up the fact that I have had my genome analyzed, and people become immediately animated, asking me about all the diseases I'm susceptible to and where they too can have a test done.

*

In an article about his feelings after having his genome scanned, Harvard psychologist Stephen Pinker (2009) wonders how much he is using the test as a means to interpret his body and his life experiences, and how much he is using his body and his life experiences to interpret his test results. He writes,

> I soon realized that I was using my knowledge of myself to make sense of the genetic readout, not the other way around. My novelty-seeking gene, for example, has been associated with a cluster of traits that includes impulsivity. But I don't think I'm particularly impulsive, so I interpret the gene as the cause of my openness to experience. But then it may be like [my] baldness gene, and say nothing about me at all.

Opening the circumference

In this book my aim has been to develop a series of conceptual and analytical tools from applied linguistics to help us understand the relationship between discourse about health and risk and the concrete social actions people take. At the crux of this relationship, I argued, are the dual processes of *entextualization* and *recontextualization* through which certain kinds of behaviors (social practices) and certain kinds of people (social identities) come to be regarded as 'healthy' or 'unhealthy', 'risky' or 'safe'. These 'technologized' social practices and social identities serve as tools for the real-time negotiation of health and risk that people engage in at various 'sites of engagement' like clinics, hospitals, health clubs, supermarkets, dinner tables, and bedrooms.

Among the most important of the texts which people appropriate to take action around health and risk, I argued, are their own bodies, and I explored the different ways people's bodies are entextualized by themselves and others by being labeled and classified, by being transformed into stories, or by being turned into artifacts like X-rays. I talked about how the texts we make of our bodies become tools not just for individual actions, but also for the promotion of larger ideological and economic agendas.

I also considered how 'cultures', communities, and social networks affect how people communicate about health and risk. I attempted to problematize traditional notions of 'culture' when it comes to research about health and risk communication, suggesting that we think not in terms of 'cultures', but in terms of 'discourse systems – systems of resources for entextualizing and recontextualizing our experiences. Everything we say, write, and do about health and risk links us to one or more discourse systems, including not just ethnic or national discourse systems, but also professional discourse systems, institutional discourse systems, gender and sexuality discourse systems, and generational discourse systems. We all participate in many overlapping discourse systems, and many of our decisions about health and risk do not arise from a unified worldview or stable set of social relationships, but rather from the need to manage multiple beliefs, multiple identities, and multiple positions *vis-à-vis* the people with whom we are interacting.

Finally, I explored how different kinds of social organizations are held together by different 'organizing discourses', and how these organizing discourses can have a profound effect on the way information and resources about health and risk are circulated throughout and across groups. I explored, for example, how communities discursively 'imagine' themselves into existence, and how sometimes these processes of imagining can have an impact on their health behavior. I also examined the organizing discourses of social networks, especially online social networks, and how they are changing the economies of knowledge and zones of expertise associated with communication about health and risk.

The most important point I wish to make in presenting this model is that, when it comes to health and risk communication, it is naïve to think that we can simply 'read off' of texts and conversations people's beliefs, actions, and experiences. When we think we can, we often find ourselves in a dilemma not unlike Pinker found himself in when reading his genetic test, not sure whether we are analyzing discourse in order to make sense of people's beliefs, actions, and experiences, or if we are analyzing people's beliefs, actions, and experiences in order to make sense of discourse. Applied linguistics, I have suggested, provides a way out of this dilemma by focusing our attention on the *tension* between the discursive resources people have available to them to take actions and form beliefs, and the strategic ways they appropriate these resources into actual social situations (Wertsch, 1994).

In their book *Nexus Analysis: Discourse and the Expanding Internet* (2004), Ron and Suzanne Scollon talk about the dangers of researchers becoming too narrowly focused on particular texts, speech events, or participants, and of the importance of learning to widen the perspective of our analysis to become conscious of how whatever text or interaction we are studying is both part of some larger social practice and connected in all sorts of complex ways to other texts, speech events, and participants. They refer to this as 'opening the circumference' of the study or, simply, 'circumferencing', which they define as 'the analytical act of opening up the angle of observation to take into consideration [the] broader discourses in which the action operates' (p. 11).

Throughout this book I have argued for 'opening the circumference' of studies of health and risk communication to explore how situated interactions such as those that take place in clinics and hospitals and everyday texts like labels on over-the-counter medications are related to larger 'discourses' through a complex interweaving of multiple 'voices', and also how these interactions and texts are part of complex chains of discourse and action that span across times, places, and people.

What this means on a practical level is that the study of health and risk communication cannot be limited to traditional 'medical settings', but must also consider what happens in places like airports, classrooms, and coffee shops. In fact, many of these interactions outside of clinics end up having a much more profound impact on our health than anything our doctor says to us. This expanded circumference would also include attention to the effects of broader social and institutional structures and ideologies and the way they might affect things like social inequalities, economic exploitation, and the marginalization of certain categories of people, issues that, as Mishler (2004) points out, are often absent in many studies of health and risk communication.

We cannot understand the impact of communication about health and risk through the analysis of discourse that has been artificially extracted from the social situations in which it occurs, or through the analysis of social situations that have been extracted from the flows of discourse and action that make up what I have been calling *discourse itineraries*. What we say and what we do is always connected to past utterances and actions and lays the ground for future ones. A true understanding of health and risk communication can only come when we start to trace the intertextual links between, for example, what a woman talks about with her doctor behind the closed door of the clinic, and what she says to her husband and children at dinner that night, the television shows she watches and the magazine articles she reads before she goes to bed, and the products that she buys in the supermarket the next day. It is in this dynamic flow of meaning, practice, and social identity that health behaviors and health beliefs are formed and changed, that communities and institutions gain or lose their influence over people, and that 'bodies of knowledge' about what it means to be healthy or sick are constructed and contested.

Applied linguistics as a *nexus of practice*

Over the past thirty years applied linguists from all corners of the field, from conversation analysis to linguistic anthropology, have engaged with issues of health and risk communication, focusing on both the micro-dynamics of situated interaction and the macro-dynamics of culture and ideology. This book has not been an attempt to present an exhaustive summary of this research or a complete description of the theoretical and analytical tools applied linguists have developed to understand health and risk communication. Indeed there is much important work I have failed to mention, many important issues I have failed to consider, and many linguistic theories and analytical tools that I have failed to describe. Rather, what I have tried to do in this book is to distil what have been for me some of the most useful concepts from applied linguistics for my own work on health and risk communication, and to integrate them into a model that others might find useful.

According to Gee (2011), a good model must always be both reflective and flexible. Being reflective means acknowledging that we as researchers are embedded in a social world, and that the way we think and talk about this world is contingent on our own professional 'storylines' and the imagined communities of scholars in which we participate. Being flexible means first of all remembering that the tools and methods we develop must change as they are adapted to specific issues, problems, and contexts, and that the models that we build are merely heuristics which make some aspects of these issues, problems, and contexts criteral and obscure others. Most importantly, being flexible means being open to insights from other disciplinary perspectives, being willing to cultivate what Sarangi (2010b, p. 413) refers to as 'analytic eclecticism'.

The principles of applied linguistics provide a way in which researchers can come to terms with these dual demands of reflexivity and flexibility. Applied linguistics is a *nexus of practice* (Scollon, 2001b) where different tools and methods from various schools of linguistics, sociology, psychology, and anthropology converge. It allows us to mold our approach to the demands of different research sites and research purposes, at one moment appropriating one set of tools (with its set of constraints and affordances) and at another moment drawing on a different set. This flexibility has become particularly important as we grapple with how to make sense of the new forms of communication, new social practices, and new kinds of social relationships made possible by new technologies.

Practical applications

It is through a wider circumference that we should also view the practical applications of our research in health and risk communication. The kind of action-oriented approach towards health and risk communication that I have advocated in this book suggests ways of improving doctor–patient communication, promoting patient 'literacy', and improving public health interventions that are very different from those traditionally pursued by scholars in health communication.

When it comes to helping doctors communicate more effectively with their patients, for example, an applied linguistic approach attempts to move beyond approaches to communication training which attempt to isolate and teach discrete 'skills' for 'effective communication' (see for example Silverman et al., 2005). Rather, it begins with a commitment to understanding the local practices of sense-making and the 'stocks of interactional knowledge' (Peräkylä and Vehviläinen, 2003) that the people we are studying already have access to. The 'major challenge of this perspective', as Frankel (1984b, p. 104) puts it, is to 'represent and understand' participants' activities 'on [their] own terms'. Applied linguistic studies of health and risk communication aim to make clear the range of functions and consequences, both positive and negative, of different textual and interactional practices (Parry, 2006). Furthermore, because their interest is in language use *in its social context*, applied linguists do not just focus on the 'inadequacies' of individual communicators, but also consider the barriers to effective communication that may result from environmental and institutional factors or from the kinds of resources people have available to them for communication. Genuinely improving interactions around health and risk requires a socially embedded, 'ecologically valid' (Cicourel, 1992) account of communication, one which captures what Sarangi and Roberts (1999, p. 2) call the 'thickly textured' and 'densely packed' nature of human activity.

Similarly, when it comes to health promotion, an applied linguistic approach does not begin with the assumption that people's 'risky' behaviors are necessarily a result of 'deficiencies' in knowledge, beliefs, attitudes, or feelings of 'self-efficacy'. Rather, it considers how behaviors arise from the ways individuals in actual interaction negotiate 'what they are doing' and 'who they are being' using the discursive resources available to them, and also how these behaviors often have their own 'local logic', sometimes functioning as strategies for individuals and groups to accomplish important social goals.

Helping people to understand and change their health and risk behaviors is often a matter of providing for them opportunities to better understand the relationship between discourse and action in their own lives. This means not just teaching them to decode the warnings on drug labels, but helping them to read texts about health and risk from drug labels to newspaper articles more critically, understanding how different processes of entextualization serve to make some aspects of an issue criterial and hide other aspects from view. It means not just teaching them to decipher entextualizations that others have made, but also giving them tools to construct their own texts, texts that can help them reflect on their behavior and formulate their own goals for changing it. Ultimately, it means helping them develop tools to address deeper issues of power and inequality in their lives and the lives of their communities and societies, tools with which, for example, they can fight for things like greater access to medical services and greater accountability from hospitals, the pharmaceutical industry, and insurance companies.

By opening the circumference of our study of health and risk communication, we begin to see the relationship between discourse and action not as just a theoretical question, but as a moral one. The wider the circumference, the more likely we are to see our work as more than just a matter of improving clinical outcomes or changing people's health behavior, but also a matter of grappling with the most fundamental questions of social justice.

REFERENCES

23andMe (2012a). 23andMe stories: Don't stand between me and my DNA. Retrieved July 12, 2012, from https://www.23andme.com/stories/1/

23andMe (2012b). 23andWe research. Retrieved July 13, 2012, from https://www.23andme.com/research/

23andMe (2012c). Terms of service. Retrieved July 13, 2012, from https://www.23andme.com/about/tos/?version=1.1

Abelson, R. P. (1976). Script processing in attitude formation and decision making. In S. John, J. S. Carroll, W. John, and J. W. Payne (Eds.), *Cognition, and Social Behavior* (pp. 33–45). Hillsdale, NJ: Lawrence Erlbaum Associates.

Ackerknecht, E. H. (1967). *Medicine at the Paris hospital, 1794–1848.* Baltimore, MD: Johns Hopkins Press.

Adam, B. D. (2005). Constructing the neoliberal sexual actor: Responsibility and care of the self in the discourse of barebackers. *Culture, Health & Sexuality, 7*(4), 333–46.

Adam, B. D. (2006). Infectious behaviour: Imputing subjectivity to HIV transmission. *Social Theory & Health, 44*(2), 168–79.

Adelswärd, V., and Sachs, L. (1998). Risk discourse: Recontextualization of numerical values in clinical practice. *Text, 18*(2), 191–210.

Adolphs, S., Atkins, S., and Harvey, K. (2007). Caught between professional requirements and interpersonal needs: Vague language in health care contexts. In J. Cutting (Ed.), *Vague language explored* (pp. 62–78). Basingstoke: Palgrave.

Ahmad, W. I. U. (Ed.). (1993). *'Race' and health in contemporary Britain.* Buckingham: Open University Press.

Ainsworth-Vaughn, N. (1998). *Claiming power in doctor–patient talk.* Oxford: Oxford University Press.

Aitken, R. C. B. (1969). Measurement of feelings using visual analogue scales. *Proceedings of the Royal Society of Medicine, 62*(10), 989–93.

Als, A. B. (1997). The desk-top computer as a magic box: Patterns of behaviour connected with the desk-top computer: GPs' and patients' perceptions. *Family Practice, 14*(1), 17–23.

American Medical Association (2001). *American Medical Association guide to talking to your doctor.* New York: Wiley.

American Medical Association (2011). *Molecular and Clinical Genetics Panel of the Medical Devices Advisory Committee: Notice of meeting [Docket No. FDA-2011-N-0066].* Retrieved July 5, 2012, from http://www.fda.gov/downloads/AdvisoryCommittees/CommitteesMeetingMaterials/

MedicalDevices/MedicalDevicesAdvisoryCommittee/MolecularandClinicalGeneticsPanel/ UCM248559.pdf.

Anderson, B. (1991). *Imagined communities: Reflections on the origin and spread of nationalism.* London: Verso.

Angelelli, C. V. (2012). Medicine. In C. B. Paulston, S. F. Kiesling, and E. S. Rangel (Eds.), *The handbook of intercultural discourse and communication* (pp. 430–48). London: Wiley Blackwell.

Armstrong, D. (1982). The doctor–patient relationship: 1930–80. In P. Wright and A. Treacher (Eds.), *The problem of medical knowledge: Examining the social construction of medicine.* Edinburgh: Edinburgh University Press.

Armstrong, D. (1983). *Political anatomy of the body: Medical knowledge in Britain in the twentieth century.* Cambridge: Cambridge University Press.

Armstrong, D. (1984). The patient's view. *Social Science & Medicine*, 18(9), 737–44.

Armstrong, D. (1995). The rise of surveillance medicine. *Sociology of Health & Illness*, 17(3), 393–404.

Aronsson, K., and Sätterlund-Larsson, U. (1987). Politeness strategies and doctor–patient communication. On the social choreography of collaborative thinking. *Journal of Language and Social Psychology*, 6(1), 1–27.

Atkinson, J. M., and Heritage, J. (1984). *Structures of social action: Studies in conversation analysis.* Cambridge: Cambridge University Press.

Atkinson, P. (1995). *Medical talk and medical work: The liturgy of the clinic.* London: Sage.

Atkinson, P. (1997). Narrative turn or blind alley? *Qualitative Health Research*, 7(3), 325–44.

Atkinson, P. (2009). Illness narratives revisited: The failure of narrative reductionism. *Sociological Research Online*, 14(5), 16.

Atkinson, P., and Silverman, D. (1997). Kundera's immortality: The interview society and the invention of the self. *Qualitative Inquiry*, 3(3), 304–25.

Austin, J. L. (1976). *How to do things with words* (2nd ed.). Oxford: Oxford University Press.

Baggaley, J. (1993). Media health campaigning: Not just what you say but the way that you say it! In A. Klusacek and K. Morrison (Eds.), *A leap in the dark: AIDS, art and contemporary cultures* (pp. 109–19). Montréal: Vehicule Press.

Baillie, C., Hewison, J., and Mason, G. (1999). Should ultrasound scanning in pregnancy be routine? *Journal of Reproductive and Infant Psychology*, 17(2), 149–57.

Bakhtin, M. M. (1981). *The dialogic imagination: Four essays* (C. Emerson and M. Holquist, Trans.). Austin, TX: University of Texas Press.

Bakhtin, M. M. (1986). *Speech genres and other late essays.* Austin, TX: University of Texas Press.

Bandura, A. (1990). Perceived self-efficacy in the exercise of control over AIDS infection. *Evaluation and Program Planning*, 13(1), 9–17.

Banks, W. P., and Thompson, S. C. (1996). The mental image of the human body: Implications of physiological mental models on our understanding of health and illness. In J. S. Mio and A. N. Katz (Eds.), *Metaphor: Implications and applications* (pp. 99–126). Mahwah, NJ: Eribaum.

Barnes, J. A. (1954). Class and committees in a Norwegian island parish. *Human Relations*, 7(1), 39–58.

Barthes, R. (1982). The photographic message. In S. Susan (Ed.), *A Barthes reader* (pp. 194–210). New York: Hill & Wang.

Barton, D., and Hamilton, M. (2005). Literacy, reification and the dynamics of social interaction. In D. Barton and K. Tusting (Eds.), *Beyond communities of practice: Language, power and social context* (pp. 14–35). Cambridge: Cambridge University Press.

Barton, E. (2004). Discourse methods and critical practice in professional communication: The front-stage and back-stage discourse of prognosis in medicine. *Journal of Business and Technical Communication*, 18(1), 67–111.

Barton, E. (2007). Institutional and professional orders of ethics in the discourse practices of research recruitment in oncology. In R. Iedema (Ed.), *The discourse of hospital communication:*

Tracing complexities in contemporary health care organizations (pp. 18–38). Basingstoke: Palgrave.

Bassett, L. (2012). Tom Corbett, Pennsylvania governor, on ultrasound mandate: Just 'close your eyes'. Retrieved March 20, 2012, from www.huffingtonpost.com/2012/03/15/tom-corbett-ultrasound-bill-pennsylvania_n_1348801.html 1/3

Bauman, R., and Briggs, C. L. (1990). Poetics and performance as critical perspectives on language and social life. *Annual Review of Anthropology*, 19, 59–88.

Beacco, J.-C., Claudel, C., Doury, M., Petit, G., and Reboul-Touré, S. (2002). Science in media and social discourse: New channels of communication, new linguistic forms. *Discourse Studies*, 4(3), 277–300.

Beach, W. A. (2001). Stability and ambiguity: Managing uncertain moments when updating news about mom's cancer. *Text*, 21(1/2), 221–50.

Beach, W. A. (2009). *A natural history of family cancer: Interactional resources for managing illness.* New York: Hampton Press.

Beck, C. S., and Ragan, S. L. (1992). Negotiating interpersonal and medical talk: Frame shifts in the gynaecologic exam. *Journal of Language and Social Psychology*, 11(1–2), 47–61.

Beck, U. (1992). *Risk Society: Towards a new modernity.* Newbury Park, NJ: Sage.

Beckman, H. B., and Frankel, R. M. (1984). The effect of physician behavior on the collection of data. *Annals of Internal Medicine*, 101(5), 692.

Beckman, H. B., Frankel, R. M., and Darnley, M. (1985). Soliciting the patient's complete agenda: A relationship to the distribution of concerns. *Clinical Research*, 33, 7174A.

Bell, C., and Newby, H. (1976). Husbands and wives: The dynamics of the deferential dialectic. In D. L. Barker and S. Allen (Eds.), *Dependence and exploitation in work and marriage* (pp. 152–68). London: Longman.

Berg, D. M., and Robb, S. (1992). Crisis management and the "paradigm case". In E. L. Toth and R. L. Heath (Eds.), *Rhetorical and critical approaches to public relations* (pp. 93–109). Hillsdale, NJ: Lawrence Erlbaum Associates.

Berg, M., and Bowker, G. (1997). The multiple bodies of the medical record: Toward a sociology of an artifact. *Sociological Quarterly*, 38(3), 513–37.

Berg, R. C., and Grimes, R. (2011). Do traditional risk factors predict whether men who have sex with men engage in unprotected anal intercourse? The need for locally based research to guide interventions. *Health*, 15(5), 517–31.

Berger, P. L., and Luckmann, T. (1967). *The social construction of reality: A treatise in the sociology of knowledge.* Garden City, NY: Doubleday.

Berkowitz, R., and Callen, M. (1983). *How to have sex in an epidemic: One approach.* New York: Tower Press.

Bhatia, V. K. (1993). *Analysing genre: Language use in professional settings.* London: Longman.

Blackburn, H. (1983). Research and demonstration projects in community cardiovascular disease prevention. *Journal of Public Health Policy*, 4(4), 398–421.

Blommaert, J. (2005). *Discourse: A critical introduction.* Cambridge: Cambridge University Press.

Bloor, M. (1995). A user's guide to contrasting theories of HIV-related risk behavior. In J. Gabe (Ed.), *Medicine, health, and risk: Sociological approaches.* Oxford: Blackwell.

Bobe, J. (2008). Biocensorship for the biocentury? Retrieved July 8, 2012, from http://thepersonalgenome.com/2008/07/biocensorship-for-the-biocentury.

Bokhour, B. G. (2006). Communication in interdisciplinary team meetings: What are we talking about? *Journal of Interprofessional Care*, 20(4), 349–63.

Bott, E. (1957). *Family and social network.* London: Tavistock Press.

Bourdieu, P. (1984). *Distinction: A social critique of the judgement of taste* (R. Nice, Trans.). Cambridge, MA: Harvard University Press.

Boyd, R. (1993). Metaphor and theory change: What is 'metaphor' a metaphor for? In A. Ortony (Ed.), *Metaphor and thought* (2nd ed., pp. 481–532). Cambridge: Cambridge University Press.

Brandt, A. M., and Rozin, P. (1997). *Morality and health.* New York: Routledge.

Brighouse, D., and Guard, B. (1992). Anaesthesia for Caesarean section in a patient with Ehlers-Danlos syndrome type IV. *British Journal of Anaesthesia*, 69(5), 517–19.

Brody, H. (1987). *Stories of sickness*. New Haven: Yale University Press.

Brown, B., Crawford, P., and Carter, R. (2006). *Evidence based health communication*. Maidenhead: Open University Press.

Brown, P., and Levinson, S. C. (1987). *Politeness: Some universals in language usage*. Cambridge: Cambridge University Press.

Brubaker, J. R., Lustig, C., and Hayes, G. R. (2010). *Patients like me: Empowerment and representation in a patient-centered social network*. Paper presented at the CSCW 2010 Workshop on CSCW Research in Healthcare: Past, Present, and Future.

Brubaker, R., and Cooper, F. (2000). Beyond "identity". *Theory and Society*, 29(1), 1–47.

Bruner, J. (1985). An historical and conceptual perspective. In J. V. Wertsch (Ed.), *Culture, communication and cognition: Vygotskian perspectives* (pp. 21–34). Cambridge: Cambridge University Press.

Buckley, W. F. (1986). Crucial steps in combating the Aids epidemic: Identify all the carriers. Retrieved December 23, 2011, from http://www.nytimes.com/books/00/07/16/specials/buckley-aids.html

Bull, S. S. (2001). HIV and sexually transmitted infection risk behaviors among men seeking sex with men on-line. *American Journal of Public Health*, 91(6), 988–89.

Bülow, P. H. (2004). Sharing experiences of contested illness by storytelling. *Discourse and Society*, 15(1), 33–53.

Burke, K. (1969). *A grammar of motives*. Berkeley, CA: University of California Press.

Bury, M. (2001). Illness narratives: Fact or fiction? *Sociology of Health and Illness*, 23(3), 263–85.

Butler, D. (2012). Canadian researcher likens controversial MS treatment to faith healing. Retrieved July 24, 2012, from http://www.canada.com/health/Canadian+researcher+likens+controversial+treatment+faith+healing/6661235/story.html.

Byrne, P. S., and Long, B. E. L. (1976). *Doctors talking to patients: A study of the verbal behaviour of general practitioners consulting in their surgeries*. Exeter: Royal College of General Practitioners.

Cain, C. (1991). Personal stories: Identity acquisition and self-understanding in alcoholics anonymous. *Ethos*, 19(2), 210–53.

Calsamiglia, H., and van Dijk, T. A. (2004). Popularization discourse and knowledge about the genome. *Discourse & Society*, 15(4), 369–89.

Cameron, R., and Williams, J. (1997). Sentence to ten cents: A case study of relevance and communicative success in nonnative–native speaker interactions in a medical setting. *Applied Linguistics*, 18(4), 415–45.

Campos, H. (2011). Hugo Campos fights for the right to open his heart's data. Retrieved July 5, 2012, from http://www.tedxcambridge.com/thrive/hugo-campos.

Candlin, C. N., and Candlin, S. (2002). Discourse, expertise, and the management of risk in health care settings. *Research on Language & Social Interaction*, 35(2), 115–37.

Candlin, C. N., and Candlin, S. (2003). Health care communication: A problematic site for applied linguistic research. *Annual Review of Applied Linguistics*, 23, 134–54.

Card, S., Mackinlay, J., and Shneiderman, B. (Eds.). (1999). *Readings in information visualization: Using vision to think*. San Francisco: Morgan Kaufmann.

Cassel, J. (1976). The contribution of the social environment to host resistance. *Am J Epidemiol*, 104(2), 107–23.

Ceng, Y., and Ren, F. (Eds.). (1997). 艾滋病 *AIDS*: 世纪的警告 (*AIDS: The warning of the century*). Beijing: People's Press.

Centers for Disease Control and Prevention (2007). *HIV/AIDS surveillance report*, Volume 17, Revised Edition, June 2007, Atlanta, GA: Centers for Disease Control and Prevention.

Černý, M. (2010). Interruptions and overlaps in doctor-patient communication revisited. Retrieved December 15, 2011, from http://www.phil.muni.cz/linguistica/art/cerny/cer-002.pdf.

Chafe, R., Born, K. B., Slutsky, A. S., and Laupacis, A. (2011). The rise of people power. *Nature*, 472(7344), 410–11.

Chandran, S., and Menon, G. (2004). When a day means more than a year: Effects of temporal framing on judgments of health risk. *Journal of Consumer Research*, 31(2), 375–89.

Charon, R. (2001). Narrative medicine: Form, function, and ethics. *Annals of Internal Medicine*, 134(1), 83–87.

Chatwin, J. (2006). Patient narratives: A micro-interactional analysis. *Communication & Medicine*, 3(2), 113–23.

Chen, R. T., and DeStefano, F. (1998). Vaccine adverse events: Causal or coincidental? *Lancet*, 351(9103), 611–12.

Chen, T. T. (2003). History of statistical thinking in medicine. In Y. Lu and J.-Q. Fang (Eds.), *Advanced medical statistics* (pp. 3–19). Singapore: World Scientific.

Chenail, R. J. (1991). *Medical discourse and systemic frames of comprehension*. Norwood, NJ: Ablex.

Cheshire, J., and Ziebland, S. (2005). Narrative as a resource in accounts of the experience of illness. In J. Thornborrow and J. Coates (Eds.), *The sociolinguistics of narrative* (pp. 17–40). Philadelphia: John Benjamins.

Chouliaraki, L., and Fairclough, N. (1999). *Discourse in late modernity: Rethinking critical discourse analysis*. Edinburgh: Edinburgh University Press.

Christakis, N. A., and Fowler, J. H. (2007). The spread of obesity in a large social network over 32 years. *The New England Journal of Medicine*, 357(4), 370–79.

Christakis, N. A., and Fowler, J. H.(2008). The collective dynamics of smoking in a large social network. *The New England Journal of Medicine*, 358(21), 2249–58.

Christakis, N. A., and Fowler, J. H. (2010). Social network sensors for early detection of contagious outbreaks. *PLoS One*, 5(9), e12948.

Cicourel, A. V. (1983). Hearing is not believing: Language and the structure of belief in medical communication. In A. Duranti and C. Goodwin (Eds.), *The social organisation of doctor–patient communication* (pp. 138–55). Washington, DC: Centre for Applied Linguistics.

Cicourel, A. V. (1992). The interpenetration of communicative contexts: Examples from medical encounters. In A. Duranti and C. Goodwin (Eds.), *Rethinking context: Language as an interactive phenomenon* (pp. 291–310). Cambridge: Cambridge University Press.

Clark, J. A., and Mishler, E. G. (1992). Attending to patients' stories: Reframing the clinical task. *Sociology of Health and Illness*, 14(3), 344–70.

Clarke, A. E., Shim, J. K., Mamo, L., Fosket, J. R., and Fishman, J. R. (2003). Biomedicalization: Technoscientific transformations of health, illness, and U.S. biomedicine. *American Sociological Review*, 68(2), 161–94.

Clatts, M. C. (1995). Disembodied acts: On the perverse use of sexual categories in the study of high-risk behaviour. In H. ten Brummelhuis and G. Herdt (Eds.), *Culture and sexual risk: Anthropological perspectives of AIDS* (pp. 241–56). Sydney: Gordon and Breach.

Clements, I., and Buczkiewicz, M. (1993). *Approaches to peer-led health education: A guide for youth workers*. London: Health Education Authority.

Cobb, S. (1976). Social support as a moderator of life stress. *Psychosomatic Medicine*, 38(5), 300–314.

Cole-Kelly, K. (1992). Illness stories and patient care in the family practice context. *Family Medicine*, 24(1), 45–48.

Conrad, P. (2007). *The medicalization of society*. Baltimore, MD: Johns Hopkins University Press.

Cook-Gumperz, J., and Messerman, L. (1999). Local identities and institutional practices: Constructing the record of professional collaboration. In S. Sarangi and C. Roberts (Eds.), *Talk, work and institutional order: Discourse in medical, mediation and management settings* (pp. 145–81). New York: Mouton de Gruyter.

Cook, G. (2004). *Genetically modified language: The discourse of arguments for GM crops and food*. London: Routledge.

Cook, G., Pieri, E., and Robbins, P. T. (2004). The scientists think and the public feels: Expert perceptions of the discourse of GM food. *Discourse & Society*, 15(4), 433–49.

Cotten, P., Lustre, N., Schimel, S., Thomas, R., and Wagner, K. (1999). *Speaking out about sex in silent spaces*. Paper presented at the The Rubberless Fuck.

Coupland, J., Robinson, J. D., and Coupland, N. (1994). Frame negotiation in doctor–elderly patient consultations. *Discourse & Society*, 5(1), 89–124.

Coupland, N., Coupland, J., and Giles, H. (1991). *Language, society and the elderly: Discourse, identity, and ageing*. Oxford: Blackwell.

Crawford, P., Brown, B., Nerlich, B., and Koteyko, N. (2008). The 'moral careers' of microbes and the rise of the matrons: An analysis of UK national press coverage of methicillin-resistant staphylococcus aureus (MRSA) 1995–2006. *Health, Risk & Society*, 10(4), 331–47.

Crawford, R. (1980). Healthism and the medicalization of everyday life. *International Journal of Health Sciences*, 10(3), 365–88.

Crichton, J., and Koch, T. (2011). Narrative, identity and care: Joint problematisation in a study of people living with dementia. In C. Candlin and J. Crichron (Eds.), *Discourses of deficit* (pp. 101–18). Houndmills: Palgrave Macmillan.

Crookshank, F. G. (1923). The importance of a theory of signs and a critique of language in the study of medicine. In C. K. Ogden and I. A. Richards (Eds.), *The meaning of meaning: A study of the influence of language upon thought and of the science of symbolism* (5th ed.). London: Routledge & Kegan Paul.

Cusick, L., and Rhodes, T. (2002). Accounting for unprotected sex: Stories of agency and acceptability. *Social Science & Medicine*, 15(2), 211–26.

Danisch, R., and Mudry, J. (2008). Is it safe to eat that? Raw oysters, risk assessment and the rhetoric of science. *Social Epistemology*, 22(2), 129–43.

Davidson, B. (2000). The interpreter as institutional gatekeeper: The socio-linguistic role of interpreters in Spanish-English medical discourse. *Journal of Sociolinguistics*, 4(3), 379–405.

Davies, B., and Harré, R. (1990). Positioning: The discursive construction of selves. *Journal for the Theory of Social Behaviour*, 20(1), 43–63.

Davison, C., and Smith, G. D. (1995). The baby and the bath water: Examining socio-cultural and free-market critiques of health promotion. In R. Bunton, S. Nettleton and R. Burrows (Eds.), *The sociology of health promotion: Critical analyses of consumption, lifestyle and risk* (pp. 91–103). London: Routledge.

Dawkins, R. (2006). *The selfish gene: 30th anniversary edition*. Oxford: Oxford University Press.

Deleuze, G., and Guattari, F. (1987). *A thousand plateaus: Capitalism and schizophrenia* (B. Massumi, Trans.). Minneapolis: University of Minnesota Press.

Dembosky, A. (2011). Invasion of the body hackers. Retrieved July 13, 2012, from www.ft.com/cms/s/2/3ccb11a0–923b-11e0–9e00–00144feab49a.html#axzz1pTueXXIL.

Denzin, N. K. (1987). *The recovering alcoholic*. Newbury Park: Sage.

DiClemente, C. C., Marinilli, A. S., Singh, B., and Bellino, E. (2000). The role of feedback in the process of health behavior change. *American Journal of Health Behavior*, 25(3), 217–27.

Diller, L. H. (2006). *The last normal child: Essays on the intersection of kids, culture,and psychiatric drugs*. Westport: Praeger.

Dolan, E. W. (2012). NOW President O'Neill: Abortion ultrasound bills are 'ritual humiliation laws'. Retrieved April 23, 2012, from http://www.rawstory.com/rs/2012/02/22/now-president-oneill-abortion-ultrasound-bills-areritual-humiliation-laws.

Donald, A., and Muthu, V. (2002). Measles. *Clinical Evidence*, 7(June), 331–40.

Donovan, J. (1984). Ethnicity and health: A research review. *Social Science and Medicine*, 19(7), 663–70.

Douglas, M. (1966). *Purity and danger: An analysis of concepts of pollution and taboo*. London: Routledge.

Douglas, M., and Calvez, M. (1990). The self as a risk-taker. *Sociological Review*, 38(3), 951–62.

Douglas, M., and Wildavsky, A. (1982). *Risk and culture: An essay on the selection of technical and environmental dangers*. Berkeley, CA: University of California Press.

Dunbar, R. (1996). *Grooming, gossip and the evolution of language*. Cambridge, MA: Harvard Univerity Press.

Dunt, D., Day, N., and Pirkis, J. (2007). Evaluation of a community-based health promotion program supporting public policy initiatives for a healthy diet. *Health Promotion International*, 14(4), 317–27.

Duranti, A. (1986). The audience as co-author: An introduction. *Text*, 6(3), 239–47.

Durkheim, E. (1952). *Suicide: A study in sociology* (J. A. Spaulding and G. Dimpson, Trans.). Glencloe, IL: The Free Press.

Edwards, D., and Potter, J. (1992). *Discursive psychology*. London: Sage.

Eggert, L. L., and Nicholas, L. J. (1992). Speaking like a skipper: 'Skippin' an' gettin' high'. *Journal of Language and Social Psychology*, 11(1–2), 75–100.

Eggly, S. (2002). Physician-patient co-construction of illness narratives in the medical interview. *Health Communication*, 14(3), 339–60.

Elwyn, G. J., and Gwyn, R. (1999). Stories we hear and stories we tell: Analysing talk in clinical practice. *British Medical Journal*, 318(7), 177–86.

English-Lueck, J. A. (2010). *Being and well-being: Health and the working bodies of Silicon Valley*. Stanford, CA: Stanford University Press.

Erickson, E. H. (1994). *Identity and the life cycle*. New York: Norton.

Erickson, F. (1996). Ethnographic microanalysis. In S. L. McKay and N. H. Hornberger (Eds.), *Sociolinguistics and language teaching* (pp. 283–306). Cambridge: Cambridge University Press.

Erickson, F., and Rittenberg, W. (1987). Topic control and person control: A thorny problem for foreign physicians in interaction with American patients. *Discourse Processes*, 10(4), 401–15.

Eriksson, N., Macpherson, J. M., Tung, J. Y., Hon, L. S., Naughton, B., Saxonov, S., et al. (2010). Web-based, participant-driven studies yield novel genetic associations for common traits. *PLoS Genet*, 6(6), e1000993.

Ertelt, S. (2012). Victory: Appeals court upholds Texas' ultrasound-abortion law. Retrieved April 23, 2012, from http://www.lifenews.com/2012/01/10/victory-appeals-court-upholds-texas-ultrasound-abortion-law.

Evans, D. A., Block, M. R., Steinberg, E. R., and Penrose, A. M. (1986). Frames and heuristics in doctor-patient discourse. *Social Science and Medicine*, 22(10), 1027–34.

Evidence-Based Medicine Working Group (1992). A new approach to teaching the practice of medicine. *Journal of the American Medical Association*, 268(17), 2420–25.

Fahy, K., and Smith, P. (1999). From the sick role to subject positions: A new approach to the medical encounter. *Health*, 3(1), 71–94.

Fairclough, N. (1989). *Language and power*. London: Longman.

Fairclough, N. (1992a). *Discourse and social change*. Oxford: Polity Press.

Fairclough, N. (Ed.). (1992b). *Critical language awareness*. Harlow: Longman.

Featherstone, M. (1991). The body in consumer culture. In M. Featherstone, M. Hepworth and B. S. Turner (Eds.), *The body: Social process and cultural theory* (pp. 170–96). London: Sage.

Fernandez-Luke, L., Elahi, N., and Grajales, F. J. (2009). An analysis of personal medical information disclosed in YouTube videos created by patients with multiple sclerosis. In K.-P. Adlassnig, B. Blobel, J. Mantas and I. Masic (Eds.), *Medical informatics in a united and healthy Europe* (pp. 292–96). Amsterdam: IOS Press.

Ferris, T. (2010). *The 4-hour body: An uncommon guide to rapid fat-loss, incredible sex, and becoming superhuman*. New York: Crown.

Finkelstein, J. (2007) *The art of self invention: Image and identity in popular visual culture*. London: I.B. Tauris & Co.

Fishbein, M., and Middlestadt, S. E. (1989). Using the theory of reasoned action as a framework for understanding in changing AIDS-related behaviors. In V. M. Mays, G. W. Albee and S. F. Schneider (Eds.), *Primary prevention of AIDS: Psychological approaches* (pp. 93–110). Newbury Park, CA: Sage.

Fisher, S. (1995). *Nursing wounds: Nurse practitioners/doctors/women patients and the negotiation of meaning*. New Brunswick, NJ: Rutgers University Press.

Fleischman, S. (1999). I am … , I have … , I suffer from … : A linguist reflects on the language of illness and disease. *Medical Humanities*, 20(1), 3–32.

Fletcher, J. C., and Evans, M. l. (1983). Maternal bonding in early fetal ultrasound examinations. *New England Journal of Medicine*, 309(2), 392–93.

Flood, M. (2003). Lust, trust and latex: Why young heterosexual men do not use condoms. *Culture, Health and Sexuality*, 5(4), 353–69.

Foster-Galasso, M. L. (2005). Diagnosis as an aid and a curse in dealing with others. In J. F. Duchan and D. Kovarsky (Eds.), *Diagnosis as cultural practice* (pp. 17–31). Berlin: Mouton de Gruyter.

Foucault, M. (1967). *Madness and civilization: A history of insanity in the age of reason*. London: Tavistock.

Foucault, M. (1972). *The archaeology of knowledge*. New York: Pantheon.

Foucault, M. (1976). *The birth of the clinic: An archaeology of medical perception*. London: Tavistock.

Foucault, M. (1978–88). *The history of sexuality* (R. Hurley, Trans. Vol. 1–3). New York: Pantheon Books.

Fox, N. J. (1993). *Postmodernism, sociology and health*. Toronto: University of Toronto Press.

Fox, S. (2011). The social life of health information, 2011. Retrieved from http://pewinternet.org/~/media//Files/Reports/2011/PIP_Social_Life_of_Health_Info.pdf.

Francis, G., and Kramer-Dahl, A. (1992). Grammaticalizing the medical case history. In M. Toolan (Ed.), *Language, text and context: Essays in stylistics* (pp. 56–92). London: Routledge.

Frank, A. W. (1995). *The wounded storyteller: Body, illness, and ethics*. Chicago: University of Chicago Press.

Frankel, R. M. (1984a). From sentence to sequence: Understanding the medical encounter through microinternational analysis. *Discourse Processes*, 7(2), 135–70.

Frankel, R. M. (1984b). Physicians and patients in social interaction: Medical encounters as a discourse process. *Discourse Processes*, 7(2), 103–5.

Frankel, R. M. (1990). Talking in interviews: A dispreference for patient-initiated questions in physician patient encounters. In G. Psathas (Ed.), *Interaction competence* (pp. 231–62). Washington, DC: University Press of America.

Frankel, R. M., Altschuler, A., George, S., Kinsman, J., Jimison, H., Robertson, N. R., et al. (2005). Effects of exam-room computing on clinician-patient communication: A longitudinal qualitative study. *Journal of General Internal Medicine*, 20(8), 677–82.

Frost, J. H., and Massagli, M. P. (2008). Social uses of personal health information within PatientsLikeMe, an online patient community: What can happen when patients have access to one another's data. *Journal Medical Internet Research*, 10(3), e15.

Frost, J. H., and Smith, B. K. (2003). *Visualizing health: Imagery in diabetes education*. Paper presented at the Designing For User Experiences.

Fry-Revere, S. (2007). When an ultra-sound becomes political. Retrieved April 15, 2012, from http://articles.chicagotribune.com/2007-05-17/news/0705160971_1_partial-birth-ultrasound-abortion.

Fung, H. (1994). The socialization of shame in young Chinese children. Unpublished doctoral dissertation. University of Chicago.

Gabe, J., and Calnan, M. (1989). The limits of medicine: Women's perception of medical technology. *Social Science & Medicine*, 28(3), 223–31.

Garfinkel, H. (1967). *Studies in ethnomethodology*. Englewood Cliffs, NJ: Prentice Hall.

Garro, L. C. (1994). Narrative representations of chronic illness experience: Cultural models of illness, mind, and body in stories concerning the temporomandibular joint (TMJ). *Social Science & Medicine*, 38(6), 775–88.

Gee, J. P. (1996). *Social linguistics and literacies: Ideology in discourses* (2nd ed.). London: Taylor & Francis.

Gee, J. P. (2003). *What video games have to teach us about learning and literacy*. Houndmills: Palgrave-MacMillan.

Gee, J. P. (2011). *An introduction to discourse analysis: Theory and method* (3rd ed.). New York: Routledge.

Gibson, G., and Copenhaver, G. P. (2010). Consent and Internet-enabled human genomics. *PLoS Genet*, 6(6), 1–5.

Giddens, A. (1979). *Central problems in social theory: Action, structure, and contradiction in social analysis*. Berkeley, CA: University of California Press.

Giddens, A. (1991). *Modernity and self-identity: Self and society in the late modern age*. Cambridge: Polity Press.

Gigerenzer, G. (2002). *Reckoning with risk: Learning to live with uncertainty*. London: Allen Lane.

Gilman, S. L. (1995). *Picturing health and illness: Images of identity and difference*. Baltimore, MD: Johns Hopkins University Press.

Goetz, T. (2007). 23AndMe will decode your DNA for $1,000. Welcome to the age of genomics. *Wired*, 15(12).

Goetz, T. (2010). *The decision tree: Taking control of your health in the new era of personalized medicine*. New York: Rodale.

Goffman, E. (1959). *The presentation of self in everyday life*. New York: Doubleday.

Goffman, E. (1961). *Asylums: Essays on the social situation of mental patients and other inmates*. New York: Anchor Books.

Goffman, E. (1963). *Stigma: Notes on the management of spoiled identity*. Englewood Cliffs, NJ: Prentice Hall.

Goffman, E. (1966). *Behavior in public places: Notes on the social organization of gatherings*. New York: The Free Press.

Goffman, E. (1974). *Frame analysis: An essay on the organization of experience*. New York: Harper and Row.

Goffman, E. (1981). *Forms of talk*. Oxford: Blackwell.

Goffman, E. (1983). The interaction order: American Sociological Association, 1982 presidential address. *American Sociological Review*, 48(1), 1–17.

Goffman, E. (1987). *Gender advertisements*. New York: Harper and Collins.

Good, B. J. (1994). *Medicine, rationality, and experience: An anthropological perspective*. Cambridge: Cambridge University Press.

Goodwin, C. (1994). Professional vision. *American Anthropologist*, 96(3), 606–33.

Greenhalgh, S. (2001). *Under the medical gaze: Facts and fictions of chronic pain*. Berkeley, CA: University of California Press.

Greenhalgh, T. (1998). Narrative based medicine in an evidence based world. In T. Greenhalgh and B. Hurwitz (Eds.), *Narrative based medicine: Dialogue and discourse in clinical practice* (pp. 247–65). London: BMJ Books.

Greenhalgh, T., and Hurwitz, B. (Eds.). (1998). *Narrative based medicine: Dialogue and discourse in general practice*. London: BMJ Books.

Greenhalgh, T., Potts, H. W. W., Gong, G., Bark, O., and Swinglehurst, D. (2009). Tensions and paradoxes in electronic patient record research: A systematic literature review using the meta-narrative method. *The Milbank Quarterly*, 87(4), 729–88.

Grinker, R. R. (2007). *Unstrange minds: Remapping the world of autism*. New York: Basic Books.

Gudelunas, D. (2012). There's an app for that: The uses and gratifications of online social networks for gay men. *Sexuality & Culture*, 14 January, 1–19.

Gumperz, J. J. (1982). *Discourse strategies*. Cambridge: Cambridge University Press.

Gumperz, J. J., and Hymes, D. (Eds.). (1964). *The ethnography of communication*. Washington, DC: American Anthropological Association.

Guttmacher Institute (2012). State policy in brief: Requirements for ultrasound. Retrieved April 30, 2012, from http://www.guttmacher.org/statecenter/spibs/spib_RFU.pdf.

Gwyn, R. (2002). *Communicating health and illness*. London: Sage.

Hacking, I. (1986). Making up people. In T. C. Heller, M. Sosna, and D. E. Wellbery (Eds.), *Reconstructing individualism: Autonomy, individuality, and the self in Western thought* (pp. 222–36). Stanford, CA: Stanford University Press.

Hak, T. (1999). "Text" and "con-text": Talk bias in studies of health care work. In S. Sarangi and C. Roberts (Eds.), *Talk, work and institutional order: Discourse in medical, mediation, and management settings* (pp. 427–52). Berlin: Mouton de Gruyter.

Halkitis, P. N., and Parsons, J. T. (2003). Intentional unsafe sex (barebacking) among HIV positive gay men who seek sexual partners on the Internet. *AIDS Care*, 15(3), 367–78.

Halkowski, T. (2006). Realizing the illness: Patients' narratives of symptom discovery. In J. Heritage and D. Maynard (Eds.), *Communication in medical care: Interaction between primary care physicians and patients* (pp. 86–114). Cambridge: Cambridge University Press.

Halliday, M. A. K. (1973). *Explorations in the functions of language*. New York: Elsevier North-Holland.

Halliday, M. A. K., and Martin, J. R. (1993). *Writing science: Literacy and discursive power.* London: Falmer Press.

Hamilton, H. E. (1998). Reported speech and survivor identity in on-line bone marrow transplantation narratives. *Journal of Sociolinguistics*, 2(1), 53–67.

Hamilton, H. E. (2003). Patients' voices in the medical world: An exploration of accounts of noncompliance. In D. Tannen and J. E. Alatis (Eds.), *Georgetown University round table on languages and linguistics 2001* (pp. 147–65). Washington, DC: Georgetown University Press.

Hamilton, H. E. (2004). Symptoms and signs in particular: The influence of the medical concern on the shape of physician-patient talk. *Communication & Medicine*, 1(1), 59–70.

Hanne, M., and Hawken, S. J. (2007). Metaphors for illness in contemporary media. *Medical Humanities*, 33(2), 93–99.

Harré, R. (2003). The discursive turn in social psychology. In D. Schiffrin, D. Tannen, and H. E. Hamilton (Eds.), *The handbook of discourse analysis* (pp. 688–706). Malden, MA: Blackwell Publishers.

Harré, R., and Moghaddam, F. M. (2003). *The self and others: Positioning individuals and groups in personal, political, and cultural contexts*. Westport, CT: Praeger.

Harrison, A., Xaba, N., and Kunene, P. (2001). Understanding safe sex: Gender narratives of HIV and pregnancy prevention by rural South African school-going youth. *Reproductive Health Matters*, 9(17), 63–71.

Hartouni, V. (1992). Fetal exposures: Abortion politics and optics of allusion. *Camera Obscura*, 10(2–28), 130–49.

Hasan, R. (1985). *Linguistics, language and verbal art*. Victoria: Deakin University.

Hauskeller, C. (2006). *Human genomics as identity politics*. Paper presented at the Young Scholar Conference Cornell University. Retrieved from from http://www.genomicsnet work.ac.uk/media/Microsoft%20Word%20-%20Identity%20Politics%20revised%20acknowl%20(2).pdf.

Haythornthwaite, C. (2009). *Online knowledge crowds and communities*. Paper presented at the International Conference on Knowledge Communities.

Heath, C. (1986). *Body movement and speech in medical interaction*. Cambridge: Cambridge University Press.

Heath, C. (1992). The delivery and reception of diagnosis in the general-practice consultation. In P. Drew and J. Heritage (Eds.), *Talk at work: Interaction in institutional settings* (pp. 235–67). Cambridge: Cambridge University Press.

Henderson, S. (2002). Consumerism in the hospital context. In S. Henderson and A. R. Petersen (Eds.), *Consuming health: The commodification of health care* (pp. 105–20). London: Routledge.

Henzl, V. M. (1989). Linguistic means of social distancing in physician-patient communication. In W. Raffler-Engel (Ed.), *Doctor–patient interaction* (pp. 77–91). Amsterdam: John Benjamins.

Herida, M., Alix, J., Devaux, I., Likatavicius, G., Desenclos, J. C., Matic, S., et al. (2007). HIV/AIDS in Europe: Epidemiological situation in 2006 and a new framework for surveillance. *Eurosurveillance*, 12(47), pii=3312.

Heritage, J. (1984). *Garfinkel and ethnomethodology*. Cambridge: Polity Press.

Heritage, J. (2005). Revisiting authority in physician-patient interaction. In J. F. Duchan and D. Kovarsky (Eds.), *Diagnosis as cultural practice* (pp. 83–102). Berlin and New York: Mouton de Gruyter.

Heritage, J., and Greatbatch, D. (1991). On the institutional character of institutional talk: The case of news interview interaction. In D. Boden and D. H. Zimmerman (Eds.), *Talk and social structure: Studies in ethnomethodology and conversation analysis* (pp. 93–137). Berkeley, CA: University of California Press.

Heritage, J., and Lindstrom, A. (1998). Motherhood, medicine, and morality: Scenes from a medical encounter. *Research on Language & Social Interaction*, 31(3–4), 397–438.

Heritage, J., and Stivers, T. (1999). Online commentary in acute medical visits: A method of shaping patient expectations. *Social Science and Medicine*, 49(11), 1501–17.

Hilbert, R. (1984). The acultural dimensions of chronic pain: Flawed reality construction and the problem of meaning. *Social Problems*, 31(4), 365–78.

Hilgartner, S. (1990). The dominant view of popularization: Conceptual problems, political uses. *Social Studies of Science*, 20(3), 519–39.

Hillman, B. J., and Goldsmith, J. C. P. (2010). The uncritical use of high-tech medical imaging. *The New England Journal of Medicine*, 363(1), 4–6.

Hobson-West, P. (2003). Understanding vaccination resistance: Moving beyond risk. *Health, Risk & Society*, 5(3), 273–83.

Hodge, B., and Louie, K. (1998). *Politics of Chinese language and culture: The art of reading dragons*. London: Routledge.

Hodge, R., and Kress, G. (1988). *Social semiotics*. Cambridge: Polity Press.

Hoey, M. (1994). Signaling in discourse: A functional analysis of a common discourse pattern in written and spoken English. In M. Coulthard (Ed.), *Advances in written text analysis* (pp. 26–45). London: Routledge.

Honeyman, A., Cox, B., and Fisher, B. (2005). Potential impacts of patient access to their electronic care records. *Informatics in Primary Care*, 13(1), 55–60.

Hull, G. A., and Katz, M. (2006). Crafting an agentive self: Case studies of digital storytelling. *Research in the Teaching of English*, 41(1), 43–81.

Humphreys, K. (2000). Community narratives and personal stories in Alcoholics Anonymous. *Journal of Community Psychology*, 28(5), 495–506.

Hunter, K. M. (1993). *Doctors' stories: The narrative structure of medical knowledge*. Princeton, NJ: Princeton University Press.

Hydén, L.-C. (1997). Illness and narrative. *Sociology of Health & Illness*, 19(1), 48–69.

Hydén, L.-C., and Bülow, P. H. (2003). Who's talking: Drawing conclusions from focus groups-some methodological considerations. *International Journal of Social Research Methodology*, 6(4), 305–21.

Hymes, D. (1974). *Foundations in sociolinguistics: An ethnographic approach*. Philadelphia: University of Pennsylvania Press.

Iedema, R. (2001a). Analyzing film and television: A social semiotic account of 'Hospital: An unhealthy business'. In T. van Leeuwen and C. Jewitt (Eds.), *Handbook of visual analysis* (pp. 183–204). London: Sage.

Iedema, R. (2001b). Resemiotization. *Semiotica*, 137(1–4), 23–39.

Iedema, R. (2003a). *Discourses of post-bureaucratic organization*. Amsterdam: John Benjamins.

Iedema, R. (2003b). The medical record as organizing discourse. *Document Design*, 4(1), 64–84.

Iedema, R. (2011). *Designing the cross professional interface: The ambulance to emergency department protocol*. Paper presented at the First Interdisciplinary Conference on Applied Linguistics and Professional Practice.

Iedema, R., Braithwaite, J., Jorm, C. M., Nugus, P., and Whelan, A. (2005). Clinical governance: Complexities and promises. In P. Stanton, E. Willis and S. Young (Eds.), *Health care reform and industrial change in Australia: Lessons, challenges and implications* (pp. 253–78). Basingstoke: Palgrave Macmillan.

Iedema, R., Rhodes, C., and Scheeres, H. (2006). Surveillance, resistance, observance: The ethics and aesthetics of identity (at) work. *Organization Studies*, 27(8), 1111–30.

Iedema, R., and Scheeres, H. (2003). From doing work to talking work: Renegotiating knowing, doing, and identity. *Applied Linguistics*, 24(3), 316–26.

Institute for the Future (2003). *Health and health care, 2010: The forecast, the challenge* (2nd ed.). San Francisco: Jossey-Bass.

Jaworski, A., and Coupland, N. (1999). Introduction: Perspectives on discourse analysis. In A. Jaworski and N. Coupland (Eds.), *The discourse reader* (pp. 1–44). London: Routledge.

Jensen, G. H. (2000). *Storytelling in alcoholics anonymous: A rhetorical analysis*. Carbondale, IL: Southern Illinois University Press.

Jewson, N. D. (1976). The disappearance of the sick-man from medical cosmology, 1770–1870. *Sociology*, 10(2), 225–44.

Jones, R. H. (1996). *Responses to AIDS awareness discourse: A cross-cultural frame analysis*. Hong Kong: Department of English, City University of Hong Kong.

Jones, R. H. (1999). Mediated action and sexual risk: Searching for 'culture' in discourses of homosexuality and AIDS prevention in China. *Culture, Health & Sexuality*, 1(2), 161–80.

Jones, R. H. (2002a). Mediated action and sexual risk: Discourses of sexuality and AIDS in the People's Republic of China. Unpublished doctoral dissertation. Macquarie University.

Jones, R. H. (2002b). A walk in the park: Frames and positions in AIDS prevention outreach among gay men in China. *Journal of Sociolinguistics*, 6(4), 575–88.

Jones, R. H. (2005a). Mediated addiction: The drug discourses of Hong Kong youth. *Health, Risk & Society*, 7(1), 25–45.

Jones, R. H. (2005b). *Sexual risk and the Internet*. Paper presented at the Language and global communication conference, Cardiff, Wales, July 7-9.

Jones, R. H. (2005c). Sites of engagement as sites of attention: Time, space and culture in electronic discourse. In S. Norris and R. H. Jones (Eds.), *Discourse in action: Introducing mediated discourse analysis* (pp. 144–54). Abingdon: Routledge.

Jones, R. H. (2007). Imagined comrades and imaginary protections: Identity, community and sexual risk among men who have sex with men in China. *Journal of Homosexuality*, 53(3), 83–115.

Jones, R. H. (2009a). Dancing, skating and sex: Action and text in the digital age. *Journal of Applied Linguistics*, 6(3), 283–302.

Jones, R. H. (2009b). Learning about AIDS online: Identity and expertise on a gay internet forum. In C. Higgins and B. Norton (Eds.), *Language and HIV/AIDS* (pp. 171–96). Bristol: Multilingual Matters.

Jones, R. H. (2011). Discourse, technology, and "bodies without organs". In C. Thurlow and K. Mroczek (Eds.), *Digital discourse: Language in the new media* (pp. 321–39). Oxford: Oxford University Press.

Jones, R. H. (2012). Constucting and consuming 'displays' in online environments. In S. Norris (Ed.), *Multimodality in practice: Investigating theory-in-practice-through-methodology* (pp. 82–96). New York: Routledge.

Jones, R. H., and Candlin, C. N. (2003). Constructing risk across timescales and trajectories: Gay men's stories of sexual encounters. *Health, Risk & Society*, 5(2), 199-213.

Jones, R. H., Candlin, C. N., and Yu, K. K. (2000). *Culture, communication and the quality of life of people living with HIV/AIDS*. Hong Kong: Council for the AIDS Trust Fund.

Jones, R. H., and Hafner, C. A. (2012). *Understanding digital literacies: A practical introduction*. London: Routledge.

Kannel, W. B., Kagan, A., Dawber, T. R., and Revotskie, N. (1962). Epidemiology of coronary heart disease: Implications for the practicing physician. *Geriatrics*, 17(Oct.), 675–90.

Katz, J. (1984). *The silent world of doctor and patient*. New York: Free Press.

Keeney, B. P. (1987). Recursive frame analysis: A method for organizing therapeutic discourse. Unpublished manuscript. Department of Human Development and Family Studies, Texas Tech University.

Kellner, D. (1992). Popular culture and the construction of postmodern identity. In S. Lash and J. Friedman (Eds.), *Modernity and identity* (pp. 141–77). Oxford: Blackwell.

Keogh, P., Beardsell, S., Davies, P., Hickson, F., and Weatherburn, P. (1998). Gay men and HIV: Community responses and personal risks. In M. T. Wright, B. R. S. Rosser and O. de Zwart (Eds.), *New international directions in HIV prevention for gay and bisexual men* (pp. 59–73). London: Harrington Park Press.

Kevles, B. H. (1997). *Naked to the bone: Medical imaging in the twentieth century*. New Brunswick, NJ: Rutgers University Press.

King, E. (1993). *Safety in numbers*. London: Cassell.

Kippax, S., Conell, R., Dowsett, G., and Crawford, J. (1993). *Sustaining safe sex: Gay communities respond to AIDS*. London: Falmer Press.

Klausner, J. D., Wolf, W., Fischer-Ponce, L., Zolt, I., and Katz, M. H. (2000). Tracing a syphilis outbreak through cyberspace. *JAMA*, 284(4), 447–49.

Kleinman, A. (1980). *Patients and healers in the context of culture: An exploration of the borderland between anthropology, medicine, and psychiatry*. Berkeley, CA: University of California Press.

Kleinman, A. (1986). *Social origins of distress and disease: Depression, neurasthenia, and pain in modern China*. New Haven: Yale University Press.

Kleinman, A. (1988). *The illness narratives: Suffering, healing, and the human condition*. New York: Basic Books.

Knudsen, S. (2003). Scientific metaphors going public. *Journal of Pragmatics*, 35(8), 1247–63.

Korsch, B. M., and Negrete, V. F. (1972). Doctor–patient communication. *Scientific American*, 227, 66–74.

Koteyko, N., and Nerlich, B. (2007). Multimodal discourse analysis of probiotic web advertising. *The International Journal of Language Society and Culture*, 23, 20–31.

Kreps, G. L., and Kunimoto, E. N. (1994). *Effective communication in multicultural healthcare settings*. Thousand Oaks, CA: Sage.

Kress, G. R. (1989). *Linguistic processes in sociocultural practice* (2nd ed.). Oxford: Oxford University Press.

Kress, G. R., and van Leeuwen, T. (1996). *Reading images: The grammar of visual design*. London: Routledge.

Kristeva, J. (1980). *Desire in language: A semiotic approach to literature and art* (T. Gora, A. Jardine and L. S. Roudiez, Trans.). New York: Columbia University Press.

Kumar, A., Hessini, L., and Mitchell, E. M. H. (2009). Conceptualising abortion stigma. *Culture, Health & Sexuality*, 11(6), 625–39.

Kutz, G. (2010). *Direct to consumer genetic tests: Misleading test results are further complicated by deceptive marketing and other questionable practices*. Washington, DC: United States Government Accountability Office.

Labov, W. and Waletzky, J. (1967) Narrative analysis: Oral versions of personal experience. J. Helm (Ed.) *Essays on the verbal and visual arts* (pp. 12-44). Seattle, WA: American Ethnological Society.

Lakoff, G., and Johnson, M. (1980). *Metaphors we live by*. Chicago: University of Chicago Press.

Lalonde, M. (1974). *A new perspective on the health of Canadians: A working document*. Ottawa: Information Canada.

Lambert, B. L., Street, R. L., Cegala, D. J., Smith, D. H., Kurtz, S., and Schofield, T. (1997). Provider-patient communication, patient-centered care, and the mangle of practice. *Health Communication*, 9(1), 27.

Landau, E. (2011). Tatoos: A journey of HIV acceptance. Retrieved 15 April, 2012, from http://edition.cnn.com/2011/HEALTH/08/10/hiv.tattoos/index.html.

Langlie, J. K. (1977). Social networks, health beliefs, and preventive health behavior. *Journal of Health and Social Behavior*, 18(3), 244–60.

Latour, B., and Woolgar, S. (1986). *Laboratory life: The construction of scientific facts*. Princeton, NJ: Princeton University Press.

Laumann, E. O., Gagnon, J. H., Michaels, S., Michael, R. T., and Coleman, J. S. (1989). Monitoring the AIDS epidemic in the U.S.: A network approach. *Science*, 244(4909), 1188–89.

Lave, J., and Wenger, E. (1991). *Situated learning: Legitimate peripheral participation*. Cambridge: Cambridge University Press.

Layder, D. (1993). *New strategies in social research*. Cambridge: Polity Press.

Lehoux, P., Poland, B., and Daudelin, G. (2006). Focus group research and "the patient's view". *Social Science & Medicine*, 63(8), 2091–2104.

Lemke, J. L. (1990). *Talking science: Language, learning, and values*. Norwood, NJ: Ablex.

Lemke, J. L. (1995). *Textual politics: Discourse and social dynamics*. London: Taylor & Francis.

Lemke, J. L. (1998). Metamedia literacy: Transforming meanings and media. In D. Reinking, M. C. McKenna, L. D. Labbo, and R. D. Kieffer (Eds.), *Handbook of literacy and technology: Transformations in a post-typographic world* (pp. 312–33). Mahwah, NJ: Lawrence Erlbaum.

Lemke, J. L. (2000). Across the scales of time: Artifacts, activities, and meanings in ecosocial systems. *Mind, Culture, and Activity*, 7(4), 273–90.

Levina, M., and Quinn, R. (2011). From symptomatic to pre-symptomatic patient: the tide of personal genomics. *Journal of Science Communication*, 10(3), C03–C07.

Levinson, S. C. (1979). Activity types and language. *Linguistics*, 17(5/6), 365–99.

Lévy, P. (1998). *Becoming virtual: Reality in the digital age* (R. Bononno, Trans.). New York: Plenum.

Li, I., Dey, A. K., and Forizzi, J. (2011). *Understanding my data, myself: Supporting selfreflection with Ubicomp technologies.* Paper presented at the UbiComp '11.

Liaw, S. T. (1993). Patient and general practitioner perceptions of patient-held health records. *Family Practice*, 10(4), 406–15.

Linell, P., Adelswärd, V., Sachs, L., Bredmar, M., and Lindstedt, U. (2002). Expert talk in medical contexts: Explicit and implicit orientation to risks. *Research on Language & Social Interaction*, 35(2), 195–218.

Løkeland, M. (2004). The legal right has been won, but not the moral right. *Reproductive Health Matters*, 12(24 Supplement), 167–73.

Lupton, D. (1995). *The imperative of health: Public health and the regulated body.* Thousand Oaks, CA: Sage.

Lupton, D. (2003). *Medicine as culture: Illness, disease and the body in Western societies* (2nd ed.). London: Sage.

Lynch, M., and Bogen, D. (1994). Harvey Sacks's primitive natural science. *Theory, Culture & Society*, 11(4), 65–104.

Ma, M., Dollar, K. M., Kibler, J. L., Sarpong, D., and Samuels, D. (2011). The effects of priming on a public health campaign targeting cardiovascular risks. *Prevention Science*, 12(3), 333–38.

Malinowski, B. (1923). The problem of meaning in primitive languages. In C. K. Ogden and I. A. Richards (Eds.), *The meaning of meaning: A study of the influence of language upon thought and of the science of symbolism* (pp. 296–336). London: Routledge.

Mangione-Smith, R., Stivers, T., Elliott, M., McDonald, L., and Heritage, J. (2003). Online commentary during the physical examination: A communication tool for avoiding inappropriate antibiotic prescribing? *Social Science and Medicine*, 56(2), 313–20.

Marcocia, M. (2004). Online polylogues: Conversation structure and participation frame work in internet newsgroups. *Journal of Pragmatics*, 36(1), 115–45.

Margalit, R. S., Roter, D., Dunevant, S. L., and Reis, S. (2006). Electronic medical record use and physician–patient communication: An observational study of Israeli primary care encounters. *Patient Education and Counseling*, 61(1), 134–41.

Martin, G. P., and Finn, R. (2011). Patients as team members: Opportunities, challenges and paradoxes of including patients in multi-professional healthcare teams. *Sociology of Health & Illness*, 33(7), 1050–65.

Marvel, M. K., Epstein, R. M., Flowers, K., and Beckman, H. B. (1999). Soliciting the patient's agenda: Have we improved? *Journal of American Medical Association*, 281(3), 283–87.

Måseide, P. (1991). Possibly abusive, often benign, and always necessary. On power and domination in medical practice. *Sociology of Health & Illness*, 13(4), 545–61.

Måseide, P. (2007a). Discourses of collaborative medical work. *Text and Talk*, 27(5/6), 611–32.

Måseide, P. (2007b). The role of signs and representations in the organization of medical work: X-rays in medical problem solving. In R. Iedema (Ed.), *The discourse of hospital communication: Tracing complexities in contemporary health care organizations* (pp. 201–21). Basingstoke: Palgrave Macmillan.

Matthews, J. R. (1995). *Quantification and the quest for medical certainty.* Princeton, NJ: Princeton University Press.

Mattingly, C., and Garro, L. C. (Eds.). (2000). *Narrative and the cultural construction of illness and healing*. Berkeley, CA: University of California Press.

Mayes, R., and Horwitz, A. V. (2005). DSM-III and the revolution in the classification of mental illness. *Journal of the History of the Behavioral Sciences*, 41(3), 249–67.

Maynard, D. W. (1991). Interaction and asymmetry in clinical discourse. *American Journal of Sociology*, 97(2), 448–95.

Maynard, D. W. (1996). On "realization" in everyday life: The forecasting of bad news as a social relation. *American Sociological Review*, 61(1), 109–31.

Maynard, D. W. (2004). On predicating a diagnosis as an attribute of a person. *Discourse Studies*, 6(1), 53–76.

McDonald, C. J. (1996). Medical heuristics: The silent adjudicators of clinical practice. *Annals of Internal Medicine*, 124(1), 56–62.

McFarlane, M., Bull, S. S., and and Rietmeijer, C. A. (2000). The internet as a newly emerging risk environment for sexually transmitted diseases. *JAMA*, 284(4), 443–46.

McGuire, A. L., and Burke, W. (2011). Health system implications of direct-to-consumer personal genome testing. *Public Health Genomics*, 14(1), 53–58.

McGuire, A. L., Diaz, C. M., Wang, T., and Hilsenbeck, S. G. (2009). Social networkers' attitudes toward direct-to-consumer personal genome testing. *American Journal of Bioethics*, 9(6–7), 3–10.

McLeroy, K. R., Norton, B. L., Kegler, M. C., Burdine, J. N., and Sumaya, C. V. (2003). Community-based interventions. *American Journal of Public Health*, 93(4), 529–33.

McNeil-PPC. (2011). New initiatives to help encourage the appropriate use of acet-aminophen. Retrieved April 8, 2012, from http://www.tylenol.com/page2.jhtml?id=tylenol/news/newdosing.inc.

Mead, G. H. (1934). *Mind, self, and society: From the standpoint of a social behaviorist*. Chicago: University of Chicago Press.

Mehan, H. (1993). Beneath the skin and between the ears: A case study in the politics of representation. In S. Chaiklin and J. Lave (Eds.), *Understanding practice: Perspectives on activity and context* (pp. 241–68). Cambridge: Cambridge University Press.

Mehta, R. (2011). The self-quantification movement. *SelfCare*, 2(3), 87–92.

Mendés-Leite, R. (1998). Imaginary protections against AIDS. In M. T. Wright, B. R. S. Rosser and O. de Zwart (Eds.), *New international directions in HIV prevention for gay and bisexual men* (pp. 103–22). London: Harrington Park Press.

Merzel, C., and D'Afflitti, J. (2003). Reconsidering community-based health promotion: Promise, performance, and potential. *American Journal of Pubiic Health*, 93(4), 557–74.

Metzger, T. A. (1981). Selfhood and authority in neo-Confucian political culture. In A. Kleinman and T. Y. Lin (Eds.), *Normal and abnormal behaviour in Chinese culture* (pp. 7–27). Dordrecht: Reidel.

Minkler, M. (1997). *Community organizing and community building for health*. New Brunswick, NJ: Rutgers University Press.

Mische, A., and White, H. (1998). Between conversation and situation: Public switching dynamics across network domains. *Social Research*, 65(3), 695–724.

Mishler, E. G. (1984). *The discourse of medicine: Dialectics of medical interviews*. Norwood, NJ: Ablex Publishing.

Mishler, E. G. (1986). *Research interviewing: Context and narrative*. Cambridge, MA: Harvard University Press.

Mishler, E. G. (1990). The struggle between the voice of medicine and the voice of the lifeworld. In P. Conrad and R. Kern (Eds.), *The sociology of health and illness: Critical perspectives* (3rd ed., pp. 295–307). New York: St. Martin's Press.

Mishler, E. G. (1995). Models of narrative analysis: A typology. *Journal of Narrative and Life History*, 5(2), 87–123.

Mishler, E. G. (1999). *Storylines: Craftartists' narratives of identity*. Cambridge, MA: Harvard University Press.

Mishler, E. G. (2004). The unjust world problem: Towards an ethics of advocacy for healthcare providers and researchers. *Communication & Medicine*, 1(1), 97–104.

Mishler, E. G., Amarasingham, L. R., Osherson, S. D., Hauser, S. T., Waxler, N. E., and Liem, R. (Eds.). (1981). *Social contexts of health, illness, and patient care*. Cambridge: Cambridge University Press.

Mitchell, L., and West, P. (1996). Peer pressure to smoke: The meaning depends on the method. *Health Education Research*, 11(1), 39–46.

Mitchell, L. M., and Georges, E. (1997). Cross-cultural cyborgs: Greek and Canadian women's discourses on fetal ultrasound. *Feminist Studies*, 23(2), 373–401.

Mitchum, P. A. (1989). Verbal and nonverbal communication in a family practice consultation: A focus on the physician-patient relationship. In W. Von Raffler-Engel (Ed.), *Doctor–Patient interaction* (pp. 109–57). Amsterdam: John Benjamins.

Mnookin, S. (2011). *The panic virus: A true story of medicine, science, and fear*. New York: Simon & Schuster.

Moirand, S. (2003). Communicative and cognitive dimensions of discourse on science in the French mass media. *Discourse Studies*, 5(2), 175–206.

Moisse, K. (2011). The YouTube cure: How social media shapes medical practice. Retrieved 31 July, 2012, from http://www.scientificamerican.com/article.cfm?id=the-youtube-cure.

Moore, A., Candlin, C. N., and Plum, G. A. (2001). Making sense of HIV-related viral load: One expert or two? *Culture, Health & Sexuality*, 3(4), 429–50.

Morris, D. B. (1998). *Illness and culture in the postmodern age*. Berkeley, CA: University of California Press.

Moses, R. A. (2000). The discourse of pharmaceutical ads. *Texas Linguistic Forum*, 44(1), 104–13.

Moynihan, R., and Cassels, A. (2005). *Selling sickness: How drug companies are turning us all into patients*. Crows Nest: Allen and Unwin.

Murphy, T. F. (1994). *Ethics in an epidemic: AIDS, morality and culture*. Berkeley, CA: University of California Press.

Mutchler, M. G. (2000). Young gay men's stories in the States: Scripts, sex, and safety in the time of AIDS. *Sexualities*, 3(1), 31–54.

Myers, G. (2003). Risk and face: A review of the six studies. *Health, Risk & Society*, 5(2), 215–20.

Navigenics (2012). Homepage. Retrieved July 30, 2012, from http://www.navigenics.com.

Nettleton, S., and Bunton, R. (1995). Sociological critiques of health promotion. In R. Bunton, S. Nettleton and R. Burrows (Eds.), *The sociology of health promotion: Critical analyses of consumption, lifestyle and risk* (pp. 41–58). London: Routledge.

Ng, B. E., Butler, L. M., Horvath, T., and Rutherford, G. W. (2011). *Population-based biomedical sexually transmitted infection control interventions for reducing HIV infection*. The Cochrane Collaboration. New York: John Wiley & Sons, Ltd.

NHS (2004). MMR: The facts. London: Department of Health.

Norris, S., and Jones, R. H. (Eds.). (2005). *Discourse in action: Introducing mediated discourse analysis*. Abingdon: Routledge.

O'Reilly, E. B. (1997). *Sobering tales: Narratives of alcoholism and recovery*. Amherst: University of Massachusetts Press.

Ochberg, F. M. (1988). Post-traumatic therapy and victims of violence. In F. M. Ochberg (Ed.), *Post-traumatic therapy and victims of violence* (pp. 3–19). New York: Brunner/Mazel.

Ochs, E. (1988). *Culture and language development: Language acquisition and socialization in a Samoan village*. New York: Cambridge University Press.

Ochs, E. (1993). Constructing social identity: A language socialization perspective. *Research on Language & Social Interaction*, 26(3), 287–306.

Ochs, E., and Shohet, M. (2006). The cultural structuring of mealtime socialization. *New Directions for Child and Adolescent Development*, 111, 35–49.

Ochs, E., Smith, R., and Taylor, C. (1989). Detective stories at dinnertime: Problem-solving through co-narration. *Cultural Dynamics*, 2(2), 238–57.

Ornstein, C. (2002, July 16). Online access to risky sex. *Los Angeles Times*. Retrieved from http://articles.latimes.com/2002/jul/26/local/me-internet26.

Page, R. E. (2012). *Stories and social media: Identities and interaction*. New York: Routledge.

Pappas, G. (1990). Some implications for the study of doctor–patient interaction. *Social Science & Medicine*, 30(2), 199–204.

Parry, R. H. (2006). Communication practices in physiotherapy: A conversation analytic study. In L. Finlay and C. Ballinger (Eds.), *Qualitative research for allied health professionals: Challenging choices* (pp. 109–24). Chichester: Wiley & Sons.

Parry, V. (2003). The art of branding a condition. *Medical Marketing and Media*, 38(5), 43–47.

Parsons, E., and Atkinson, P. (1992). Lay constructions of genetic risk. *Sociology of Health & Illness*, 14(4), 437–55.

Parsons, T. (1951). *The social system*. New York: Free Press.

Patel, V. L., Arocha, J. F., and Kushniruk, A. W. (2002). Patients' and physicians' understanding of health and biomedical concepts: Relationship to the design of EMR systems. *Journal of Biomedical Informatics*, 35(1), 8–16.

Patel, V. L., Kushniruk, A. W., Yang, S., and Yale, J. F. (2000). Impact of a computerized patient record system of medical data collection, organization and reasoning. *JAMIA 2000*, 7(6), 569–85.

Patton, C. (1990). *Inventing AIDS*. New York: Routledge.

Patton, C. (1991). Safe sex and the pornographic vernacular. In Bad Object-Choices (Ed.), *How do I look?: Queer film and video* (pp. 31–63). Seattle: Bay Press.

Paugh, A., and Izquierdo, C. (2009). Why is this a battle every night?: Negotiating food and eating in American dinnertime interaction. *Journal of Linguistic Anthropology*, 19(2), 185–204.

Payer, L. (1992). *Disease-Mongers*. New York: John Wiley.

Pearce, C., Trumble, S., Arnold, M., Dwan, K., and Phillips, C. (2008a). Computers in the new consultation: Within the first minute. *Family Practice*, 25(3), 202–8.

Pearce, C., Walker, H., and O'Shea, C. (2008b). A visual study of computers on doctors' desks. *Informatics in Primary Care*, 16(2), 111–17.

Peräkylä, A. (1998). Authority and accountability: The delivery of diagnosis in primary health care. *Social Psychology Quarterly*, 61(4), 301–20.

Peräkylä, A. (2002). Agency and authority: Extended responses to diagnostic statements in primary care encounters. *Research on Language & Social Interaction*, 35(2), 219–47.

Peräkylä, A., Ruusuvuori, J., and Vehviläinen, S. (2005). Introduction: Professional theories and institutional interaction. *Communication and Medicine*, 2(2), 105–9.

Peräkylä, A., and Vehviläinen, S. (2003). Conversation analysis and the professional stocks of interactional knowledge. *Discourse & Society*, 14(6), 727–50.

Perry, C. L. (1989). Prevention of alcohol use and abuse in adolescents: Teachers versus peer led intervention. *Crisis*, 10(1), 52–61.

Perry, C. L., and Sieving, R. (1993). *Peer involvement in global AIDS prevention among adolescents*. Geneva: University of Minnesota/World Health Organisation.

Petchesky, R. P. (1987). Fetal images: The power of visual culture in the politics of reproduction. *Feminist Studies*, 13(2), 263–92.

Petersen, A., and Lupton, D. (1996). *The new public health: Health and self in the age of risk*. London: Sage.

Phillips, N., Lawrence, T. B., and Hardy, C. (2004). Discourse and institutions. *Academy of Management Review*, 29(4), 635–52.

Pickering, A. (1995). *The mangle of practice: Time, agency, and science*. Chicago: University of Chicago Press.

Pinker, S. (2009). My genome, myself. *New York Times Magazine*. Retrieved May 13, 2012, from www.nytimes.com/2009/01/11/magazine/11Genome-t.html?pagewanted=all.

Pisani, E. (2008). *The wisdom of whores: Bureaucrats, brothels and the business of AIDS*. London: Granta.

Plumridge, E., and Chetwynd, J. (1999). Identity and the social construction of risk: Injecting drug use. *Sociology of Health & Illness*, 21(3), 329–43.

Poirier, S., and Brauner, D. (1990). The voices of the medical record. *Theoretical Medicine*, 11(1), 23–39.

Poland, B., and Holmes, D. (2009). Celebrating risk: The politics of self-branding, transgression and resistance in public health. *Aporia*, 1(4), 27–36.

Polkinghorne, D. E. (1988). *Narrative knowing and the human sciences.* Albany, NY: State University of New York Press.

Pollack, A. (2010, June 11). FDA faults companies on unapproved genetic tests. *The New York Times.*

Pomerantz, A., Gill, V. T., and Denvir, P. (2007). When patients present serious health conditions as unlikely: Managing potentially conflicting issues and constraints. In A. Hepburn and S. Wiggins (Eds.), *Discursive research in practice: New approaches to psychology and interaction* (pp. 127–46). Cambridge: Cambridge University Press.

Porter, T. M. (1996). *Trust in numbers: The pursuit of objectivity in science and public life.* Princeton, NJ: Princeton University Press.

Potter, J., Wetherell, M., and Chitty, A. (1991). Quantification rhetoric – Cancer on television. *Discourse & Society,* 2(3), 333–65.

Prainsack, B., Reardon, J., Hindmarsh, R., Gottweis, H., Naue, U., and Lunshof, J. E. (2008). Misdirected precaution. *Nature,* 456(6), 34–35.

Prior, L. (2000). Reflections on the 'mortal' body in late modernity. In S. J. Williams, J. Gabe and M. Calnan (Eds.), *Health, medicine and society: Key theories, future agendas* (pp. 186–202). London: Routledge.

Radley, A., and Billig, M. (1996). Accounts of health and illness: Dilemmas and representations. *Sociology of Health and Illness,* 18(2), 220–40.

Rainie, L., and Wellman, B. (2012). *Networked: The new social operating system.* Cambridge, MA: MIT Press.

Rainville, S. (2009). Undeniable risks: A critical discourse analysis of the 23andMe website. Unpublished MA Dissertation. Carleton University.

Ramsay, M. E., Yarwood, J., Lewis, D., Campbell, H., and White, J. M. (2002). Parental confidence in measles, mumps and rubella vaccine: Evidence from vaccine coverage and attitudinal surveys. *British Journal of General Practice,* 52(484), 912–16.

Reddy, M. C., Dourish, P., and Pratt, A. (2001). *Coordinating hetero-geneous work: Information and representation in medical care.* Paper presented at the Proceedings of European Conference on Computer Supported Cooperative Work (ECSCCW'01).

Reisfield, G. M., and Wilson, G. R. (2004). Use of metaphor in the discourse on cancer. *Journal of Clinical Oncology,* 22(19), 4024–27.

Rhodes, T. (1994). HIV outreach, peer education and community change: developments and dilemmas. *Health Education Journal,* 53(1), 92–99.

Rhodes, T. (1997). Risk theory in epidemic times: Sex, drugs and the social organisation of 'risk behaviour'. *Sociology of Health & Illness,* 19(2), 208–27.

Richardson, K. (2003). Health risks on the internet: Establishing credibility online. *Health, Risk and Society,* 5(2), 171–84.

Riessman, C. K. (1990). Strategic uses of narrative in the presentation of self and illness. *Social Science and Medicine,* 30(11), 1195–1200.

Riessman, C. K. (1993). *Narrative analysis.* Newbury Park, CA: Sage.

Rifkin, E., Bouwer, E., and Sheff, B. (2006). *The illusion of certainty: Health benefits and risks.* New York: Springer.

Roberts, C. (2006). Continuities and discontinuities in doctor-patient consultations in a multilingual society. In M. Gotti and F. Salager-Meyer (Eds.), *Advances in medical discourse analysis: Oral and written contexts* (pp. 177–95). Bern: Peter Lang.

Roberts, C. (2010). Intercultural communication in healthcare settings. In D. Matsumoto (Ed.), *APA handbook of intercultural communication* (pp. 213–28). New York: Walter de Gruyter.

Roberts, C., Moss, B., Wass, V., Sarangi, S., and Jones, R. (2005). Misunderstandings: A qualitative study of primary care consultations in multilingual settings, and educational implications. *Medical Education,* 39(5), 465–75.

Roberts, C., Sarangi, S., and Moss, B. (2004). Presentation of self and symptom in primary care consultations involving patients from non-English speaking backgrounds. *Communication and Medicine,* 1(2), 159–69.

Roberts, F. D. (1999). *Talking about treatment: Recommendations for breast cancer adjuvant treatment.* New York: Oxford University Press.

Roberts, J. (2012). 'Wakey wakey baby': Narrating four-dimensional (4D) bonding scans. *Sociology of Health & Illness,* 34(2), 299–314.

Rose, N., and Novas, C. (2005). Biological citizenship. In A. Ong and S. Collier (Eds.), *Global assemblages: Technology, politics and ethics as anthropological problems* (pp. 439–63). London: Blackwell.

Rosenthal, D., Gifford, S., and Moore, S. (1998). Safe sex or safe love: Competing discourses? *AIDS Care,* 10(1), 34–46.

Roter, D. L., and Hall, J. A. (1992). *Doctors talking with patients/patients talking with doctors: Improving communication in medical visits.* Westport, CT: Auburn House.

Rothstein, W. G. (2003). *Public health and the risk factor: A history of an uneven medical revolution.* Rochester, NY: University of Rochester Press.

Rumelhart, D. E. (1975). Notes on a schema for stories. In D. G. Bobrow and A. Collins (Eds.), *Representation and understanding: Studies in cognitive science* (pp. 185–210). New York: Academic Press.

Sacks, H. (1967). The search for help: No one to turn to. In E. S. Shneidman (Ed.), *Essays in self destruction* (pp. 203–23). New York: Science House.

Sacks, H. (1972). An initial investigation of the usability of conversational data for doing sociology. In D. Sudnow (Ed.), *Studies in social interaction* (pp. 31–74). New York: Free Press.

Sacks, H. (1995). *Lectures on conversation.* Oxford: Blackwell.

Sacks, H., Schegloff, E. A., and Jefferson, G. (1974). A simplest systematics for the organization of turn-taking for conversation. *Language,* 50(4), 696–735.

Sacks, O. W. (1985). *The man who mistook his wife for a hat and other clinical tales.* New York: Simon & Schuster.

Sandelowski, M. (2002). Reembodying qualitative inquiry. *Qualitative Health Research,* 12(1), 104–15.

Sanders, L. (1956). *Every patient tells a story: Medical mysteries and the art of diagnosis.* New York: Basic Books.

Sarangi, S. (2000). Activity types, discourse types and interactional hybridity: The case of genetic counselling. In S. Sarangi and M. Coulthard (Eds.), *Discourse and social life* (pp. 1–27). London: Longman.

Sarangi, S. (2004). Towards a communicative mentality in medical and healthcare practice. *Communication & Medicine,* 1(1), 1–11.

Sarangi, S. (2010a). Healthcare interaction as an expert communicative system: An activity analysis perspective. In J. Streeck (Ed.), *New adventures in language and interaction* (pp. 167–98). Amsterdam: John Benjamins.

Sarangi, S. (2010b). Practising discourse analysis in healthcare settings. In I. Bourgeault, R. Dingwall and R. de Vries (Eds.), *The Sage handbook of qualitative methods in health research* (pp. 397–416). London: Sage.

Sarangi, S., Bennert, K., Howell, L., Clarke, A., Harper, P., and Gray, J. (2004). Initiation of reflective frames in counseling for Huntington's Disease predictive testing. *Journal of Genetic Counseling,* 13(2), 135–55.

Sarangi, S., and Candlin, C. N. (2003). Categorization and explanation of risk: A discourse analytical perspective. *Health, Risk & Society,* 5(2), 115–24.

Sarangi, S., and Clarke, A. (2002). Zones of expertise and the management of uncertainty in genetics risk communication. *Research on Language & Social Interaction,* 35(2), 139–71.

Sarangi, S., and Roberts, C. (1999). Introduction: The dynamics of interactional and institutional orders in work-related settings. In S. Sarangi and C. Roberts (Eds.), *Talk, work and the institutional order: Discourse in medical, mediation and management settings* (pp. 1–57). Berlin: Mouton de Gruyter.

Sarasohn-Kahn, J. (2008). *The wisdom of patients: Health care meets online social media.* Oakland, CA: California HealthCare Foundation.

Schank, R. C., and Abelson, R. P. (1977). *Scripts, plans, goals and understanding: An enquiry into human knowledge structures*. Hillsdale, NJ: Lawrence Erlbaum.

Schegloff, E. A. (1968). Sequencing in conversational openings. *American Anthropologist*, 70(6), 1075–95.

Schegloff, E. A. (1987). Some sources of understanding in talk-in-interaction. *Linguistics*, 25(1), 201–18.

Schiffrin, D. (1988). *Discourse markers*. Cambridge: Cambridge University Press.

Schiffrin, D. (1996). Narrative as self-portrait: Sociolinguistic constructions of identity. *Language in Society*, 25(2), 167–203.

Schofield, M. J., Redman, S., and Sanson-Fisher, R. W. (1991). A community approach to smoking prevention: A review. *Behaviour Change*, 8(1), 17–25.

Schwartz, L. M., and Woloshin, S. (1999). Changing disease definitions: Implications for disease prevalence. *Effective Clinical Practice*, 2(2), 76–85.

Scollon, R. (1998). *Mediated discourse as social interaction: A study of news discourse*. London: Longman.

Scollon, R. (2001a). Action and text: Towards an integrated understanding of the place of text in social (inter)action, mediated discourse analysis and the problem of social action. In R. Wodak and M. Meyer (Eds.), *Methods of critical discourse analysis* (pp. 139–83). London: Sage.

Scollon, R. (2001b). *Mediated discourse: The nexus of practice*. Oxford: Routledge.

Scollon, R. (2008). Discourse itineraries: Nine processes of resemiotization. In V. K. Bhatia, J. Flowerdew and R. H. Jones (Eds.), *Advances in discourse studies* (pp. 233–44). London: Routledge.

Scollon, R., and Scollon, S. W. (1981). *Narrative, literacy, and face in interethnic communication*. Norwood, NJ: Ablex Publishing Corporation.

Scollon, R., and Scollon, S. W. (2004). *Nexus analysis: Discourse and the emerging internet*. London: Routledge.

Scollon, R., Scollon, S. W., and Jones, R. H. (2012). *Intercultural communication: A discourse approach* (3rd ed.). Chichester: Wiley-Blackwell.

Shernoff, M. (2006). *Without condoms: Unprotected sex, gay men and barebacking*. New York: Routledge.

Shilling, C. (1993). *The body and social theory*. Newbury Park: Sage.

Silverman, D. (1987). *Communication and medical practice: Social relations in the clinic*. London: Sage.

Silverman, D. (1997). *Discourses of counselling: HIV counselling as social interaction*. London: Sage.

Silverman, D., and Peräkylä, A. (1990). AIDS counselling: The interactional organisation of talk about 'delicate' issues. *Sociology of Health & Illness*, 12(3), 293–318.

Silverman, J., Kurtz, S., and Draper, J. (2005). *Skills for communicating with patients* (2nd ed.). Abingdon: Radcliffe Medical Press.

Simmel, G. (1955). *Conflict and the web of group affiliations* (R. Bendix, Trans.). Glencoe, IL: Free Press.

Skrabanek, P. (1994). *The death of humane medicine: And the rise of coercive healthism*. Bury Saint Edmunds: Social Affairs Unit, St. Edmundsbury Press.

Slade, D., Scheeres, H., Manidis, M., Iedema, R., Dunston, R., Stein-Parbury, J., et al. (2008). Emergency communication: The discursive challenges facing emergency clinicians and patients in hospital emergency departments. *Discourse & Communication*, 2(3), 271–98.

Smith, D. H. (1999). What Hong Kong patients want and expect from their doctors. *Health Communication*, 11(3), 299–310.

Smith, M. J., Ellenberg, S. S., Bell, L. M., and Rubin, D. M. (2008). Media coverage of the measles-mumps-rubella vaccine and autism controversy and its relationship to MMR immunization rates in the United States. *Pediatrics*, 121(4), e836–e843.

Smith, M. R. (2012). Informed consent laws: Protecting a woman's right to know. *Defending life 2012*. Retrieved from http://www.aul.org/wp-content/uploads/2012/04/informed-consent-laws.pdf.

Sobo, E. J. (1995). *Choosing unsafe sex: AIDS-risk denial among disadvantaged women*. Philadelphia, PA: University of Pennsylvania Press.

Solly, M. (2007). 'Don't get caught out': Pragmatic and discourse features of informational and promotional texts in international healthcare insurance. *Communication and Medicine*, 4(1), 27–35.

Sontag, S. (1991). *Illness as metaphor and AIDS and its metaphors*. London: Penguin.

Speers, T., and Lewis, J. (2004). Journalists and jabs: Media coverage of the MMR vaccine. *Communication & Medicine*, 1(2), 171–81.

Spindler, A. (1993). Patterns. Retrieved 23 November, 2012, from http://www.nytimes.com/1993/11/23/news/patterns-214493.html?pagewanted=all&src=pm.

Stabile, A. (1992). Shooting the mother: Fetal photography and the politics of disappearance. *Camera Obscura*, 10(1–28), 179–206.

Staiano, K. V. (1986). *Interpreting signs of illness. A case study in medical semiotics*. Berlin: Mouton de Gruyter.

Star, S. L., and Greisemer, J. (1989). Institutional ecology, "translations," and boundary objects: Amateurs and professionals in Berkeley's Museum of Vertebrate Zoology, 1907–39. *Social Studies of Science*, 19(3), 387–420.

Starr, P. (1982). *The social transformation of American medicine*. New York: Basic Books.

Stivers, T., and Heritage, J. (2001). Breaking the sequential mold: Answering 'more than the question' during comprehensive history taking. *Text*, 21(1/2), 151–85.

Stommel, W. (2009). *Entering an online support group on eating disorders: A discourse analysis (Utrecht studies in language and communication)*. Amsterdam: Rodopi.

Straus, R. (1957). The nature and status of medical sociology. *American Sociological Review*, 22(2), 200–204.

Strong, P. M. (2001). *The ceremonial order of the clinic: Parents, doctors and medical bureaucracies*. Aldershot: Ashgate.

Sudnow, D. (1967). *Passing on: The social organization of dying*. Englewood Cliffs, NJ: Prentice-Hall.

Suhardja, I. (2009). The discourse of 'distortion' and health and medical news reports: A genre analysis perspective. Unpublished doctoral dissertation. University of Edinburgh.

Swales, J. M. (1990). *Genre analysis: English in academic and research settings*. Cambridge: Cambridge University Press.

Swan, M. (2009). Emerging patient-driven health care models: An examination of health social networks, consumer personalized medicine and quantified self-tracking. *International Journal of Environmental Research and Public Health*, 6(2), 492–525.

Swinglehurst, D., Roberts, C., and Greenhalgh, T. (2011). Opening up the "black box" of the electronic patient record: A linguistic ethnographic study in general practice. *Communication and Medicine*, 8(1), 3–15.

Tadele, G. (2010). "Boundaries of Sexual Safety": Men Who Have Sex with Men (MSM) and HIV/AIDS in Addis Ababa. *Journal of HIV/AIDS & Social Services*, 9, 261–80.

Tajfel, H., and Turner, J. C. (1986). The social identity theory of inter-group behavior. In W. G. Austin and S. Worchel (Eds.), *Psychology of intergroup relations* (pp. 7–24). Chicago: Nelson-Hall.

Tannen, D. (1980). A comparative analysis of oral narrative strategies: Athenian Greek and American English. In W. L. Chafe (Ed.), *The pear stories: Cognitive, cultural, and linguistic aspects of narrative production* (pp. 51–87). Norwood, NJ: Ablex Publishing.

Tannen, D. (1993). What's in a frame? Surface evidence for underlying expectations. In D. Tannen (Ed.), *Framing in discourse* (pp. 14–56). New York: Oxford University Press.

Tannen, D. (2005). *Conversational style: Analyzing talk among friends* (2nd ed.). New York: Oxford University Press.

Tannen, D. (Ed.). (1982). *Spoken and written language: Exploring orality and literacy*. Norwood, NJ: Ablex Publishing.

Tannen, D., and Wallat, C. (1987). Interactive frames and knowledge schemas in interaction: Examples from a medical examination/interview. *Social Psychology Quarterly*, 50(2), 205–16.

ten Have, P. (1989). The consultation as a genre. In B. Torode (Ed.), *Text and talk as social practice: Discourse difference and division in speech and writing* (pp. 115–35). Dordrecht: Foris Publications.

ten Have, P. (1991). Talk and institution: A reconsideration of the 'asymmetry' of doctor-patient interaction. In D. Boden and D. H. Zimmerman (Eds.), *Talk and social structure: Studies in ethnomethodology and conversation analysis* (pp. 138–63). Cambridge: Polity Press.

ten Have, P. (1995). Medical ethnomethodology: An overview. *Human Studies*, 18(2), 245–61.

Todd, A. D. (1984). The prescription of contraception: Negotiations between doctors and patients. *Discourse Processes*, 7(2), 171–200.

Todd, A. D., and Fisher, S. (Eds.). (1993). *The social organization of doctor-patient communication*. Norwood, NJ: Ablex Publishing.

Topol, E. (2012). *The creative destruction of medicine: How the digital revolution will create better health care*. New York: Basic Books.

Torrey, T. (2011). A story of misdiagnosis. How a wrong diagnosis became a source of motivation. Retrieved 23 April, 2011, from http://patients.about.com/od/misdiagnosis/a/misdiagnosis.htm.

Treichler, P. A. (1988a). AIDS, gender and biomedical discourse: Current contests for meaning. In E. Fee and D. M. Fox (Eds.), *AIDS: The burdens of history* (pp. 190–266). Berkeley, CA: University of California Press.

Treichler, P. A. (1988b). AIDS, homophobia and biomedical discourse: An epidemic of signification. In D. Crimp (Ed.), *AIDS: Cultural analysis, cultural activism* (pp. 31–70). Cambridge, MA: MIT Press.

Trudeau, G. (2012). Doonsbury. Retrieved April 30, 2012, from http://doonesbury.slate.com/strip/archive/2012/03/12.

Turner, B. S. (1984). *The body and society: Explorations in social theory*. Oxford: Basil Blackwell.

Turner, B. S. (1992). *Regulating bodies: Essays in medical sociology*. London: Routledge.

Tutton, R., and Prainsack, B. (2011). Enterprising or altruistic selves? Making up research subjects in genetics research. *Sociology of Health & Illness*, 33(7), 1081–95.

U.S. Food and Drug Administration (2012). FDA safety communication: Chronic cerebrospinal venous insufficiency treatment in multiple sclerosis patients. Retrieved July 25, 2012, from http://www.fda.gov/MedicalDevices/Safety/AlertsandNotices/ucm303318.htm.

Udéhn, L. (2001). *Methodological individualism: Background, history and meaning*. London: Routledge.

van Dijck, J. (2005). *The transparent body: A cultural analysis of medical imaging*. Seattle, WA: University of Washington Press.

van Dijk, T. A. (1993). Principles of critical discourse analysis. *Discourse & Society*, 4(2), 249–83.

van Dijk, T. A. (2003). Specialized discourse and knowledge: A case study of the discourse of modern genetics. In E. M. Morato, A. C. Bentes, M. L. C. Lima and I. G. V. Koch (Eds.), *Homenagem a Ingedore Koch* (pp. 21-56). Campinas: Departamento de Lingüística do Instituto de Estudos da Linguagem de UNICAMP.

van Dijk, T. A. (2008). *Discourse and context: A sociocognitive approach*. Cambridge: Cambridge University Press.

Van Langenhove, L., and Harré, R. (1999). Introducing positioning theory. In R. Harré and L. Van Langenhove (Eds.), *Positioning theory: Moral contexts of intentional action*. Oxford: Blackwell.

van Leeuwen, T. (1996). The representation of social actors. In C. R. Caldas-Coulthard and M. Coulthard (Eds.), *Texts and practices: Readings in critical discourse analysis* (pp. 32–70). London: Routledge.

van Ommen, G. B., and Cornel, M. C. (2008). Recreational genomics? Dreams and fears on genetic susceptibility screening. *Eur J Hum Genet*, 16(4), 403–4.

van Rijn-van Tongeren, G. W. (1997). *Metaphors in medical texts*. Amsterdam: Rodopi.

Ventres, W., Kooienga, S., Marlin, R., Vuckovic, N., and Stewart, V. (2005). Clinician style and examination room computers: A video ethnography. *Family Medicine*, 37(4), 276–81.

Vestergaard, M., Hviid, A., Madsen, K. M., Wohlfahrt, J., Thorsen, P., Schendel, D., et al. (2004). MMR vaccination and febrile seizures: Evaluation of susceptible subgroups and long-term prognosis. *Journal of American Medical Association*, 292(3), 351–57.

Vicdan, H., and Dholakia, N. (2013). Medicine 2.0 and beyond: From information seeking to knowledge creation in virtual health communities. In R. W. Belk and R. Llamas (Eds.), *The Routledge companion to digital consumption*. London: Routledge.

Voysey, M. (2006). *A constant burden: The reconstitution of family life* (2nd ed.). Aldershot: Ashgate.

Vygotsky, L. S. (1962). *Thought and language* (E. Hanfmann and G. Vakar, Trans.). Cambridge, MA: MIT Press.

Vygotsky, L. S. (1987). *The collected works of L.S. Vygotsky* (N. Minick, Trans.). New York: Plenum Press.

Wakefield, A. J. (1998). Autism, inflammatory bowel disease, and MMR vaccine (correspondence: author's reply). *The Lancet*, 351(9106), 908.

Wakefield, A. J., Murch, S. H., Anthony, A., Linnell, J., Casson, D. M., Malik, M., et al. (1998). Ileal-lymphoid-nodular hyperplasia, non-specific colitis, and pervasive developmental disorder in children. *Lancet*, 351(9103), 637–41.

Walsh, S. H. (2004). The clinician's perspective on electronic health records and how they can affect patient care. *British Medical Journal*, 328(7449), 1184–87.

Watkins, S. C., Swindler, A., and Biruk, C. (2008). Hearsay ethnography: Conversational journals as a method for studying culture in action. *California Center for Population Research, UC Los Angeles*. Retrieved from http://escholarship.org/uc/item/0hp8m602.

Watney, S. (1989). *Policing desire: Pornography, AIDS and the media*. Minneapolis, MN: University of Minnesota Press.

Watney, S. (1990). Safer sex as community practice. In P. Aggleton, P. Davies and G. Hart (Eds.), *AIDS: Individual, cultural and policy dimensions* (pp. 19–33). London: The Falmer Press.

Watney, S. (1993). Emergent sexual identities and HIV/AIDS. In P. Aggleton, P. Davies and G. Hart (Eds.), *AIDS: Facing the second decade* (pp. 13–27). London: Falmer Press.

Weingart, P. (1998). Science and the media. *Research Policy*, 27(8), 869–79.

Wertsch, J. V. (1994). The primacy of mediated action in sociocultural studies. *Mind, Culture, and Activity*, 1(4), 202–8.

Wertsch, J. V. (2001). Vygotsky and Bakhtin on community. In U. S. Larsson (Ed.), *Socio-cultural theory and methods: An anthology*. Trollhättan: University Trollhättan/Uddevalla.

West, C. (1984). *Routine complications: Troubles with talk between doctors and patients*. Bloomington: Indiana University Press.

Wing, L., and Potter, D. (2002). The epidemiology of autistic spectrum disorders: Is the prevalence rising? *Mental Retardation and Developmental Disabilities Research Reviews*, 8(3), 151–61.

Winthereik, B. R. (2004). Connecting Practices: An electronic patient record at work in primary health care. Unpublished doctoral dissertation. Erasmus University.

Wodak, R. (1996). *Disorders of discourse*. London: Longman.

Wolf, G. (2010). The data driven life. Retrieved July 15, 2012, from http://www.nytimes.com/2010/05/02/magazine/02self-measurement-t.html?pagewanted=all.

Wong, D. L., and Baker, C. M. (1988). Pain in children: Comparison of assessment scales. *Pediatric Nursing*, 14(1), 9–17.

Wright, P. (1999). Writing information design on healthcare materials. In C. N. Candlin and K. Hyland (Eds.), *Writing: Texts, processes and practices* (pp. 85–98). London: Longman.

Yanoff, K. L. (1988). *The rhetoric of medical discourse: An analysis of the major genres*. Unpublished doctoral dissertation, University of Pennsylvania, Philadelphia.

Young, J. C., and Garro, L. C. (1993). *Medical choice in a Mexican village*. Prospect Heights, IL: Waveland Press.

Young, K. (1989). Narrative embodiments: Enclaves of self in the realm of medicine. In J. Shotter and K. J. Gergen (Eds.), *Texts of identity* (pp. 152–65). London: Sage.

Zimmerman, D. H. (1998). Identity, context and interaction. In C. Antaki and S. Widdicombe (Eds.), *Identities in talk* (pp. 87–106). London: Sage.

INDEX